NEUROLOGY – LABORATORY AND CLINICAL
RESEARCH DEVELOPMENTS

RECENT DEVELOPMENTS IN NEURODEGENERATION

NEUROLOGY – LABORATORY AND CLINICAL RESEARCH DEVELOPMENTS

Additional books and e-books in this series can be found on Nova's website under the Series tab.

NEUROLOGY – LABORATORY AND CLINICAL
RESEARCH DEVELOPMENTS

RECENT DEVELOPMENTS IN NEURODEGENERATION

ROGER M. HOWE
EDITOR

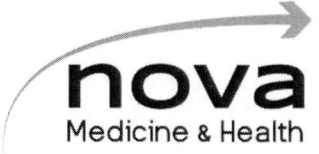

Copyright © 2020 by Nova Science Publishers, Inc.

All rights reserved. No part of this book may be reproduced, stored in a retrieval system or transmitted in any form or by any means: electronic, electrostatic, magnetic, tape, mechanical photocopying, recording or otherwise without the written permission of the Publisher.

We have partnered with Copyright Clearance Center to make it easy for you to obtain permissions to reuse content from this publication. Simply navigate to this publication's page on Nova's website and locate the "Get Permission" button below the title description. This button is linked directly to the title's permission page on copyright.com. Alternatively, you can visit copyright.com and search by title, ISBN, or ISSN.

For further questions about using the service on copyright.com, please contact:
Copyright Clearance Center
Phone: +1-(978) 750-8400   Fax: +1-(978) 750-4470   E-mail: info@copyright.com.

NOTICE TO THE READER

The Publisher has taken reasonable care in the preparation of this book, but makes no expressed or implied warranty of any kind and assumes no responsibility for any errors or omissions. No liability is assumed for incidental or consequential damages in connection with or arising out of information contained in this book. The Publisher shall not be liable for any special, consequential, or exemplary damages resulting, in whole or in part, from the readers' use of, or reliance upon, this material. Any parts of this book based on government reports are so indicated and copyright is claimed for those parts to the extent applicable to compilations of such works.

Independent verification should be sought for any data, advice or recommendations contained in this book. In addition, no responsibility is assumed by the Publisher for any injury and/or damage to persons or property arising from any methods, products, instructions, ideas or otherwise contained in this publication.

This publication is designed to provide accurate and authoritative information with regard to the subject matter covered herein. It is sold with the clear understanding that the Publisher is not engaged in rendering legal or any other professional services. If legal or any other expert assistance is required, the services of a competent person should be sought. FROM A DECLARATION OF PARTICIPANTS JOINTLY ADOPTED BY A COMMITTEE OF THE AMERICAN BAR ASSOCIATION AND A COMMITTEE OF PUBLISHERS.

Additional color graphics may be available in the e-book version of this book.

Library of Congress Cataloging-in-Publication Data

ISBN: 978-1-53618-859-2

Published by Nova Science Publishers, Inc. † New York

CONTENTS

Preface		vii
Chapter 1	Nitric Oxide and Cellular Homeostasis: Updates in Neurodegenerative Mechanisms *Parul Gupta, Abhishek Singh, Shubhangini Tiwari and Sarika Singh*	1
Chapter 2	Participation of Brain Ischemia in the Development of the Genotype and Phenotype of Alzheimer's Disease *Ryszard Pluta and Marzena Ułamek-Kozioł*	39
Chapter 3	Inflammatory Response, Excitotoxicity and Oxidative Stress Following Traumatic Brain Injury *Marco Aurelio M. Freire and Daniel Falcao*	73

Chapter 4	All Around the Nose of Parkinsonism and Essential Tremor	95
	Michael G. Sadovsky, Vladislav G. Abramov, Denis D. Pokhabov, Maria E. Tunik, Alina A. Khoroshavina, Ksenia O. Tutsenko, Tatiana B. Kovaleva, Natalia V. Malchik and Dmitry V. Pokhabov	
Index		**145**

PREFACE

Recent Developments in Neurodegeneration discusses the diverse functions of nitric oxide regarding redox regulation, the cellular energy pool, modifications in genetic material, neurogenesis, the effects on protein degradation mechanisms and functional consociation with glial cells.

The authors consider the latest evidence that demonstrates that Alzheimer's disease-associated proteins and their genes play a key role in the post-ischemic development of neurodegeneration with dementia.

The main processes associated with secondary tissue damage following traumatic injury to the nervous system are reviewed.

In closing, a comprehensive investigation of the combination of tremor and olfactory perception characteristics among patients with Parkinson's disease and essential tremor is presented.

Chapter 1 - Nitric oxide (NO) is a versatile diffusible neurotransmitter participates in various physiological and pathological mechanisms depending on its cellular levels. Particular concentration of NO is required for the physiological functions however augmented level of NO exhibits the diverse pathological mechanisms including altered cellular redox regulation, dysfunctional mitochondria and modification in genetic material. It could also execute post translational modifications in protein through S-nitrosylation of their thiol amino acids and critically affect the cellular physiology. Besides oxidative modifications NO could also nitrosylate the sensors of endoplasmic reticulum (ER) stress and consequently affect the protein degradation mechanism of cell. Such phenomenon leads to accumulation of misfolded proteins in cell forming protein aggregates. These protein aggregates are recognized as the pathological hallmarks in most of the age related central nervous system - neurodegenerative diseases including Alzheimer's, Parkinson's, Huntington's and Amyotrophic lateral sclerosis. In this chapter the authors are discussing about the diverse functions of NO involving redox regulation, cellular energy pool, modifications in genetic material, neurogenesis, effect on protein degradation mechanisms and their functional consociation with glial cells. These all NO mediated mechanisms must be taken in to account during discovery and development of therapeutics for said neurodegenerative diseases.

Chapter 2 - Transient ischemia-reperfusion brain injury generated a massive neuronal loss in the CA1 area of the hippocampus, associated with neuroinflammation. This was accompanied by progressive atrophy of the hippocampus, cerebral cortex and white matter lesions. Furthermore, it was noted that neurodegenerative post-ischemic processes continued well beyond the acute stage. Rarefaction of white matter was significantly increased in animals within 2 years post-ischemia. Some rats that survived 2 years post-ischemia developed severe brain atrophy with dementia, which indicates active and slowly progressing neurodegeneration process. The profile of post-ischemic brain neurodegeneration shares a commonality with neurodegenerative processes in Alzheimer's disease. What is even more, ischemic brain damage is associated with the accumulation of folding proteins, such as amyloid and tau protein, in the intra- and extracellular space of cells. Here, post-ischemic alterations of protein which are connected with Alzheimer's disease and changes of their genes (*amyloid protein precursor* and *tau protein*) are presented. Recent advances in understanding post-ischemic neurodegeneration have revealed dysregulation of Alzheimer's disease associated genes such as: *amyloid protein precursor, α-secretase, β-secretase, presenilin 1* and *presenilin 2,* and *tau protein*. In this chapter, the latest evidence demonstrates that Alzheimer's disease-associated proteins and their genes play a key role in post-ischemic development of neurodegeneration with dementia. Ongoing interest in brain ischemia research has provided data showing that ischemia may be involved in the development of neurodegeneration of Alzheimer's disease genotype and phenotype, suggesting that brain ischemia can be considered as a useful model for understanding processes responsible for the induction of Alzheimer's disease.

Chapter 3 - Traumatic brain injury (TBI) is a major public health problem affecting both industrialized and developing countries worldwide. It is estimated that globally, 69 million people are affected by TBI every year. The World Health Organization predicted TBI would become a worldwide leading cause of death and disability, surpassing many other diseases and treading to be the third leading cause of death worldwide by this year, 2020. The effects of TBI result in growing health and social-economic burden impacting societies throughout the world, especially low-income groups. The long-term psychosocial outcomes that follow a traumatic brain injury event generate not only an impact on the quality of life of the survivors but also directly affect the lives of caretakers, and the whole family involved. TBI knowledge has significantly increased, therefore leading to an evolving definition, better clinical categorization, and raising public awareness. Molecular and cellular processes involved with TBI have remained the focus of studies attempting to better understand associated neurochemical and metabolic responses. Recently, several studies investigating acute neural disorders due to both primary and secondary tissue damage following TBI have emerged. Following the primary trauma, which causes irreversible loss of tissue in the wounded area, the main secondary pathological mechanisms involve the physiological alteration in the levels of glutamate in the affected neural parenchyma that lead to excitotoxicity, inflammatory response, oxidative stress with subsequent disturbances in normal neurophysiological functions and ultimately cell death. Furthermore, studies have demonstrated that components of the inflammatory response are associated with both glial breakdown and demyelination, which are related to the increase of the functional deficits following the acute injury. This chapter aims to review the main processes associated with secondary tissue damage following traumatic injury to the nervous system. The understanding of the mechanisms related to neural tissue loss after TBI is crucial for the development of effective therapies that may help to minimize the debilitating condition experienced by the survivors.

Chapter 4 - The authors present comprehensive investigation of the combination of tremor and olfactory perception characteristics among the patients with Parkinson's disease and essential tremor. Tremor studies bring abundant data records and the most informative have been found. Tremor data itself fail to discriminate Parkinson's disease patients from essential tremor ones; same is true for discrimination between the sick patients and control group. The combination of tremor data and olfactory dysfunction measurements was found to improve the discrimination all groups of patients. To measure the olfactory dysfunction, the authors used Sniffin' sticks test. It was found that the standard protocol makes the olfactory data measurements biased. To avoid the bias, the authors changed the protocol through the randomization of the sticks with different smells and different agent concentrations. Randomization seriously improved the data. Besides, two other subtests had been improved. The third subtest (identification) requires an implementation of unbiased and reliable reference of the smell recalling, while the standard protocol does not do it. The authors have carried out special investigation of the unattended knowledge of smells among patients suffering from neurodegeneration, conditionally healthy persons, and those with severe trauma. These data provides the reference set of smells (and numbers of answers, as well) to improve the third Sniffin' sticks subtest. Finally, the new hypothesis towards the inverse dependence between olfactory dysfunction and tremor is proven. This fact opens new horizons in understanding of relationship between tremor and olfactory dysfunction in developments of neurodegenerative disorders. Some further progress in olfactory measurements with respect to COVID-19 infection is discussed.

In: Recent Developments in Neurodegeneration ISBN: 978-1-53618-859-2
Editor: Roger M. Howe © 2020 Nova Science Publishers, Inc.

Chapter 1

NITRIC OXIDE AND CELLULAR HOMEOSTASIS: UPDATES IN NEURODEGENERATIVE MECHANISMS

Parul Gupta, Abhishek Singh,
Shubhangini Tiwari and Sarika Singh[*]
Department of Neurosciences and Ageing Biology,
Division of Toxicology and Experimental Medicine,
CSIR-Central Drug Research Institute,
Lucknow, UP, India

ABSTRACT

Nitric oxide (NO) is a versatile diffusible neurotransmitter participates in various physiological and pathological mechanisms depending on its cellular levels. Particular concentration of NO is required for the physiological functions however augmented level of NO exhibits the diverse pathological mechanisms including altered cellular redox regulation, dysfunctional mitochondria and modification in genetic material. It could also execute post translational modifications in protein

---

[*] Corresponding Author's Email: sarika_singh@cdri.res.in; ssj3010@gmail.com.

through S-nitrosylation of their thiol amino acids and critically affect the cellular physiology. Besides oxidative modifications NO could also nitrosylate the sensors of endoplasmic reticulum (ER) stress and consequently affect the protein degradation mechanism of cell. Such phenomenon leads to accumulation of misfolded proteins in cell forming protein aggregates. These protein aggregates are recognized as the pathological hallmarks in most of the age related central nervous system - neurodegenerative diseases including Alzheimer's, Parkinson's, Huntington's and Amyotrophic lateral sclerosis. In this chapter we are discussing about the diverse functions of NO involving redox regulation, cellular energy pool, modifications in genetic material, neurogenesis, effect on protein degradation mechanisms and their functional consociation with glial cells. These all NO mediated mechanisms must be taken in to account during discovery and development of therapeutics for said neurodegenerative diseases.

Keywords: neurodegenerative diseases, nitric oxide, redox regulation, energy crisis, endoplasmic reticulum stress, unfolded protein responses, cellular homeostasis, protein aggregation, central nervous system

ABBREVIATIONS

NO	Nitric oxide
ER	Endoplasmic reticulum
AD	Alzheimer's Disease
PD	Parkinson's Disease
HD	Huntington's Disease
ALS	Amyotrophic lateral sclerosis
nNOS	Neuronal nitric oxide synthase
CNS	Central nervous system
NMDA	N-methyl-D-Aspartate
AMPA	α-amino-3-hydroxy-5-methyl-4-isoxazolepropionic acid
ROS	Reactive oxygen species
RNS	Reactive nitrogen species
GSH	reduced glutathione
SOD	superoxide dismutase

GFAP	Glial fibrillary acidic protein
LTP	long-term-potentiation
SNO	S-nitrosothiol
PDI	protein disulfide isomerase
ERAD	ER stress associated degradation
SERCA	sarcoplasmic/endoplasmic reticulum Ca^{+2}-ATPase
IRE-1	inositol-requiring enzyme 1
ATF-6	Activating Transcription Factor 6
PERK	PRKR-like endoplasmic reticulum kinase
UPR	unfolded protein response
PARP	poly (ADP-ribose) polymerase
CACT	carnitine/acyl carnitine transporter
PTEN	Phosphatase and tensin homolog
ONOO	peroxynitrite
VLCAD	very long-chain acyl-CoA dehydrogenase
L-NAME	N(G)-nitro-L-arginine methyl ester
MPTP	(1-methyl-4-phenyl-1,2,3,6-tetrahydropyridine)
GAPDH	Glyceraldehyde 3-phosphate dehydrogenase
NOS	Nitric oxide synthase
CREB	cAMP response element-binding protein
mTORC1	mammalian target of rapamycin complex 1
IKKβ	inhibitor of nuclear factor kappa-B kinase
APP	amyloid precursor protein
BACE1	beta-site amyloid precursor protein cleaving enzyme 1
H_2O_2	hydrogen peroxides

1. INTRODUCTION

Nitric oxide (NO) is a gaseous neurotransmitter synthesized from L-arginine and molecular oxygen through any one of the isoforms among three NO synthases (NOS), named as neuronal (nNOS), endothelial (eNOS), and inducible (iNOS). NO has been widely consented as a signaling molecule involved in various physiological mechanisms. Research in last two-three decades have suggested that NO has wide role in both peripheral and central nervous system (CNS). This review is focusing on the NO related pathological mechanisms involved in neurodegenerative diseases of CNS. At its physiological level NO contributes in various functions, their differentiation and survival of neurons mediated through various signaling pathways (Zhang et al., 2017; Singh, 2020) however its augmented level is critically involved in various neuropathological mechanisms as reported in different neurodegenerative diseases like Alzheimer's, Parkinson's, Huntington's and amytrophic lateral sclerosis (Sobrevia et al., 2016). The vast network of NO mediated signaling pathways includes modifications of proteins and DNA involving acetylation/deacetylation, methylation/ demethylation and nitrotyrosination of protein residues as well as modulation of gene expression via epigenetic changes (Vasudevan et al., 2016). Nitrotyrosination of proteins is done through formation of NO mediated peroxynitrite (Pacher et al., 2007). Along with modifications of proteins and genetic material, NO is also able to impair the cell function and executed the energy crisis through inhibited mitochondrial complexes activity. Previous reports have shown the inhibitory effect of NO on mitochondrial complexes though the inhibition may be reversible or irreversible depending on the component of electron transport chain (Brown, 1999; Nisoli and Carruba, 2006). NO mediated energy crisis directed the cell towards death pathway which may be of apoptotic, necrotic or autophagic which depends on the level of NO, type of cell and also on the antioxidant capability of affected cell. Excitotoxicity is another major pathologic process in most of the neurodegenerative diseases in which neurons are damaged/died due to the over activation of receptors for the excitatory neurotransmitter glutamate like N-methyl-D-Aspartate (NMDA) and α-amino-3-hydroxy-5-methyl-4-isoxazolepropionic acid (AMPA) (Beal, 1998). Excitotoxicity mainly arises with a massive release of glutamate which is well reported in all of the discussed neurodegenerative diseases (Ribeiro et al., 2017; Lau and Tymianski, 2010). Excessive activation of NMDA and AMPA receptors through excitatory amino acids leads to diverse injurious outcome including altered calcium homeostasis, generation of reactive oxygen species (ROS) and reactive nitrogen species (RNS), formation of mitochondrial transition pores through decreased mitochondrial membrane potential and secondary excitotoxicity (Doble, 1999; Dong et al., 2009). In view of previous reports, the excitotoxicity could be consider as common pathogenic event in all of the discussed neurodegenerative diseases. Epigenetic effect of NO may contribute in protein aggregation dependent hypothesis of neurodegenerative mechanisms and should be explored thoroughly. Since protein synthesis and processing takes place in endoplasmic reticulum (ER) the functionality of ER during disease onset is considerable. In this regard we and others have reported that ER stress is one of the cardinal components in disease related neuropathological mechanisms (Prentice et al., 2015; Biswas et al., 2018; Goswami et al. 2014; Gupta et al., 2019). In the subsequent sections we are discussing the NO mediated specific pathological event and major observations and evidences during pathology of neurodegenerative diseases.

2. NO Mediated Neurodegenerative Mechanisms

2.1. Nitric Oxide and Oxidative Stress

Most of the neurodegenerative diseases are age related which itself is characterized by shrunken brain area, impairment of cognitive and motor functions and formation of abnormal protein aggregates (Cenini et al., 2019). Both oxidative and nitrosative stress increase during ageing due to the high consumption of glucose and oxygen by neuronal cells to compensate for the high energy requirements in the CNS, leading to the initiation of redox reactions and production of ROS/ RNS (Rizor et al., 2019). During physiological conditions, astrocytes play a significant role in production of antioxidants such as GSH peroxidase, SOD and catalase in order to maintain the redox balance within the brain. However, pathological state marks the onset of a condition called reactive astrogliosis, characterized by upregulation of GFAP and vimentin, increased expression of glutamate transporters, overproduction of ROS/RNS species and proinflammatory cytokines which conjointly cause neurotoxicity and neuronal damage (Booth et al., 2017). The release of NO by reactive astrocytes induces lipid peroxidation, mitochondrial dysfunction and DNA damage which aggravate the cell death signaling factors and neuronal death (Tiesmann and Schulz, 2004). ROS species such as superoxide, nitric monoxide and hydroxyl ions are produced as a byproduct of oxygen metabolism and ATP production during oxidative phosphorylation and play essential role in age related various downstream cellular signaling mechanisms (Rizor et al., 2019). In brain the homeostasis of metal ions involving iron, copper and zinc is essential for its physiological functions which get easily oxidized in such oxidative environment (Umeno et al., 2017). During physiological condition, the production of ROS/RNS species remain regulated with the antioxidant capacity of neurons as well as with the production of antioxidants by the astrocytes which kept the perfect equilibrium to brain environment. However during pathological state condition, the production of ROS/RNS species is elevated and transcends the scavenging capacity of antioxidants buffer system, leading to oxidative stress including oxidative DNA lesions in the CNS (Baillet et al., 2010). Overproduction of NO and its interaction with superoxide ions produces more toxic RNS species $ONOO^-$ (Beal, 1998) which lead to increased calcium influx, ROS generation and aberrant S-nitrosylation of proteins, along with simultaneous decrease in GSH levels, facilitating oxidative/nitrosative stress, reactive astrogliosis and neurodegeneration (Hardy et al., 2018).

2.2. Nitric Oxide and Mitochondrial Dysfunction

Mitochondria are the main organelle that maintain the bioenergetics and metabolism within a neuron to perform various physiological functions specifically synaptic communication. Dysfunctional mitochondrion is linked to various neurological disorders such as Alzheimer's disease (AD), Parkinson's disease (PD), amyotrophic lateral sclerosis (ALS), ischemia and Huntington's disease (HD) (Ghasemi et al., 2018). Upregulation of iNOS and nNOS in brain during pathologic conditions and consequent generation of excessive RNS species contributes to both ageing and neuronal death, a phenomenon directly linked with mitochondria functionality (Pollard et al., 2016). NO directly or indirectly participates in the redox balance, calcium homeostasis, mitochondrial protein quality control and gene regulation to modify its function (Stepien et al., 2017). NO is able to inhibit the component of electron transport chain (ETC) of mitochondria and directly interferes in the energy status of neurons (Tengan and Moraes, 2017). Such NO mediated inhibition may be reversible or irreversible. NO bind to cytochrome c oxidase, affect the ETC and mitochondrion functionally (Hashemy et al., 2007). Aberrant NO signaling also leads to disrupted synaptic function and cause mitochondrial anomaly. S-nitrosylation of key enzymes in mitochondrial complex impairs the respiratory chain and ATP generation (Nakamura and Lipton, 2019). For example, NO nitrosylate the enzymes which are associated with TCA cycle including aconitase, α-ketoglutarate dehydrogenase, succinate, fumarate, malate and thus significantly affect the cellular NADH and ATP levels (Nakamura and Lipton, 2019). Physiological levels of NO offers S-nitrosylation of very long-chain acyl-CoA dehydrogenase (VLCAD) to promote β-oxidation of fatty acid however, increased NO levels lead to S-nitrosylation of carnitine/acyl carnitine transporter (CACT), disrupting the physiological signaling pathway and inducing toxicity in the mitochondria of neuron (Doulias et al., 2013; Tonazzi et al., 2017). S-nitrosylated Drp1 protein has been reported in postmortem brains of AD which enhances mitochondrial fragmentation, loss of synapse, dysfunctional mitochondria and neuronal death (Cho et al., 2009) validating the NO mediated nitrosylation of mitochondrial proteins. NO also play a role in mitochondrial dynamics and mitophagy and readers may read the referred article (Nakamura and Lipton, 2019). Increased NO levels directly correlate with fragmentation of mitochondria which then processed through autophagosomes for their removal. nNOS is recruited by Phosphatase and tensin homolog (PTEN) induced kinase 1 (PINK1) to the mitochondria which then maintains optimal level of NO in order to translocate the Parkin to mitochondria and induce mitophagy (Tiwari and Singh, 2020; Han et al., 2015). Anomalous PINK1 modification at C568 through S-nitrosylation inhibits the translocation of Parkin and impedes mitophagy grounds disease pathogenesis (Oh et al.,

2017). NO also S-nitrosylates the Parkin which inhibits its E3 ubiquitin activity and prevents the ubiquitination of DRP1, a substrate protein promoting high levels of DRP1 and increased during mitochondrial fragmentation (Zhang et al., 2016) signifying the role of NO in modulation of mitochondrial function, dynamics and mitochondrial vitality leading to neuronal death.

2.3. Nitric Oxide and Protein Modification

NO acts as a vasodilator which is activated due to production of cyclic GMP (cGMP) and subsequently cGMP dependent protein kinase (PKG1), responsible for smooth muscle relaxation through regulation of intracellular calcium reserves (Tegeder, 2018). In brain, neuronal NOS1-NO-cGMP-PKG1 pathway increases the release of synaptic vesicles thus neurotransmitters to support the long-term-potentiation (LTP) upon NMDA receptor activation (Bradley and Steinert, 2016). Although LTP acts in memory formation, the up regulated level of NO affects the cellular signaling which further enhances the risk of glutamate excitoxicity and summate the RNS production (Luo et al., 2012). To prevent such excitotoxicity, NO transforms the NMDA receptor, through reversible post-translational redox modification such as S-nitrosylation [S-nitrosothiol (SNO)] of cysteine residues (Kim et al., 1999). In addition to NMDA, SNO-targets include various other proteins which are related to maintenance of neuronal function involving calmodulin, caspase3, Glyceraldehyde 3-phosphate dehydrogenase (GAPDH), Nitric oxide synthase (NOS), cAMP response element-binding protein (CREB), p53 and protein disulfide isomerase (PDI) (Tegeder, 2018). Elevated generation of RNS species during various neurodegenerative diseases, cause aberrant S-nitrosylation of specific proteins on the cysteine residues not similar to those residues targeted during physiological conditions and consequently disturb the neuronal networks, synaptic function and initiate cell death signaling cascade (Nakamura et al., 2019). NO could also nitrosylate the various cellular chaperon like Heat shock proteins 70 (HSP70), HSP90, calreticulin thus affects the protein processing (Tegeder, 2018; Pratt et al., 2010). Since ER organelle is responsible for the protein synthesis and processing, the increased level of NO affect the ER functionality. PDIs are overexpressed during neuronal stress and regulate protein maturation and transport of proteins to protect against neuronal injury (Walker et al., 2009). S-nitrosylation of PDI severely hampers its thiol-sulfide oxidoreductase based catalytic functions, which leads to aggregation of proteins executing ER stress associated degradation (ERAD), proteosome dysfunction, autophagy and neuronal death (Tiwari and Singh, 2020). Aberrant association of SNO on the enzymatic sites of PINK1 and DRP1 severely compromises the mitochondrial activity, bioenergetics and protein quality control. Post translational modification (nitration) by peroxynitrite on the tyrosine residue of target proteins in mitochondria also hampers the mitochondrial functions and contributes to disease pathogenesis (Nakamura et al., 2019). Nitration of α-synuclein, β-amyloid and Tau leads to their aggregation and accumulation in the neuron marking the onset of disease pathology (Giasson et al., 2000; Kummur et al., 2011; Reynolds et al., 2005). Transnitrosylation is a phenomenon that occurs due to transfer of SNO group from one protein (transnitrosylating) to another (denitrosylating) protein. SNO-caspase3 and XIAP participate in transnitrosylation reaction wherein SNO group is transferred from caspase3 to XIAP which inhibits its anti-apoptotic property and reactivates cleaved caspase3 after denitrosylation which exacerbates the neuronal death mechanisms (Nakamura et al., 2010). nNOS is upregulated in the ageing brain suggestive of stress mechanisms and dysfunctional protein quality check. Persistent generation of RNS species and high levels of NO also contribute to ageing, promote protein misfolding as observed in α- synucleinopathy, taupathy, aggregation of β-amyloid and mutant huntingtin, majorly accepted hallmarks of various age related neurodegenerative diseases.

2.4. Nitric Oxide and Endoplasmic Reticulum Stress

ER serves to maintain calcium homeostasis by pumping Ca^{+2} in to the ER lumen via sarcoplasmic/endoplasmic reticulum Ca^{+2}-ATPase (SERCA) and release of Ca^{+2} from ER (Schroder et al., 2005). High Ca^{+2} is required for the physiological function of ER and protein folding with the presence of ER chaperons like calreticulin, calnexin and PDI. Among various ER chaperons calreticulin and calnexin members contribute in protein quality control system and may participate in the synthesis of glycosylated proteins. NO being free radical nitrosylate the ER chaperons thus cause disruption in Ca^{+2} homeostasis and consequent impaired physiological functions of ER. Such impaired ER functionality caused accumulation of misfolded proteins in ER (Oyadomari et al., 2001). High levels of NO and impaired ER functions initiate the apoptotic signaling (Oyadomari et al., 2002). Initial state of functional impairment of ER endeavor to overcome such stress by activating the ER membrane located transmembrane kinases (IRE-1, ATF-6 and PERK), also called as ER sensor and attempt to attenuate the translation and prevent the accumulation of unfolded protein and unfolded protein responses (UPRs) (Gupta et al., 2020; Chu et al., 2019, Ghemrawi et al., 2020). However due to increased level of NO, the chaperons get nitrosylated and could not perform their physiological function and unfolded/misfolded protein accumulate in the ER lumen, where misfolded or unfolded proteins are further recognized by the molecular named as PDI. Molecular chaperones may participate important role in maintenance of protein quality control and recover from the stress. Under the normal or moderate accumulation of misfolded protein in ER lumen the UPRs initiate to overcome ER stress by inhibiting the further protein translation or activates the molecular chaperons like GRP-78/Bip and PDI to restore ER function. NO also nitrosylates the transmembrane protein kinase like PERK and IRE-1 and nitrosylation of PERK induces the kinase activity that could participate to regulate the protein translation by phosphorylation of eIF2α and nitrosylation of IRE-1which also affects the splicing activity of XBP-1 that promotes the expression of gene related neuroprotective effects (Nakato et al., 2015, Tiwari et al., 2020). It was also reported that the depletion in the

Ca^{+2} due to nitrosylation also induces the ER stress by activation of ATF-6 and GADD153 in the cells (Oyadomari et al., 2002).

2.5. Nitric Oxide and Protein Degradation Mechanism

After translation the proteins translocated to the ER lumen for their proper folding to attain their native and physiological stable structure. Functional impairment of ER lead to misfolding or unfolding of proteins which consequently accumulate in the ER lumen and physiologically could be degraded by ER chaperons. Degradation of unfolded or misfolded proteins occurs via the proteasomal degradation machinery. Proteasome is a multiprotein complex made up of 20S core and 19S regulatory units and degrades the proteins through proteolysis (Tai and Schuman 2008, Asano et al., 2015). Augmented level of NO could S-nitrosylate the proteins which could not perform their physiological functions and must be degraded from the cellular system (Uehara et al., 2006). Such nitosylated proteins could be degraded by proteasome machinery with involvement of chaperons mainly HSPs like HSP60, HSP70 and HSP90 which require ATP for their action (Saibil et al., 2013) and may also involve master regulator of chaperone mediated autophagy (CMA) and ubiquitin -2 ligase UBE2D (Tekirdag et al., 2017). It has also been reported that iNOS could also be degraded by proteasome machinery (Musial and Eissa, 2001) therefore suggesting that increased level of NO and depleted proteasome machinery could be one of the reasons behind neurodegenerative signalling during neurodegenerative diseases. It has also been suggested that ubiquitination is essentially required for degradation of iNOS by proteasome machinery (Kolodziejski et al., 2002) suggesting that depleted proteasome activity during neurodegenerative disease may be one of the reasons behind augmented activity of iNOS and increased level of NO however studies are required for substantiation of direct association. However, NO mediated regulation of proteasome machinery during neurodegradation has been suggested (Bal et al., 2017) and further detailed investigations are required.

2.6. Nitric Oxide and DNA Damage

Exogenous exposure of the NO and their metabolites causes direct or indirect genotoxic effects. NO actively interacts with the oxygen to form nitrosating agents like nitrous ion, NOX, N_2O_3 which could modify the cellular DNA and may cause its impaired functionality (Singh, 2020). In last few years the significant involvement of NO signaling has been suggested in epigenetics however the functional association during health and disease remain to be studied (Socco et al., 2017). NO has also been emerged as a key player which mediates the epigenetic modifications associated with cell cycle arrest and neuronal differentiation (Nott and Riccio, 2009). NO actively react with molecular oxygen to form the more toxic species peroxynitrite which induce the DNA damage through oxidation, deamination of the nitrogenous DNA bases, DNA strand break or interstrand crosslinks (Ahmad et al., 2019). DNA base that contains exocyclic amino group undergoes to deamination due to NO attack. DNA base like adenine, cytosine, 5-methylcytosine and guanine undergoes deamination to form hypoxanthine, uracil, thymine and xanthine respectively. These modifications in DNA lead to the formation of abasic sites which can be cleared by endonuclease to cause single strand breaks in DNA (Chen et al., 2001). Consequences of deamination of these DNA bases varies from nucleoside to nucleoside that causes mispairing of nucleoside base which induces instability in DNA structure and induces mutations in DNA pairing like transversion of G:C to T:A and transition of G:C To A:T (Loeb et al., 1986). NO exposures to the DNA can also leads to the formation of single strand breaks in DNA as NO directly reacts with the sugar moiety of the DNA. Damage in the sugar moiety leads to the damage in the sugar phosphate backbone of the DNA and consequent break in single strand of the DNA and mutation in the complimentary strand of the DNA. NO can also interfere in the DNA repair enzyme activity as it nitrosylate the cysteine residues in the active site of the enzymes that mainly involved in DNA ligation thus resulting in partial or complete loss of enzymatic activity. NO may also participate in kinase activity of signaling cascade, that modulates during DNA repair mechanism (Singh et al., 2013). NO also induces the

DNA damage through the induction of p53 and activation of poly (ADP-ribose) polymerase (PARP). This upregulated p53 blocked the cellular proliferation during cell cycle phase G1 checkpoint or induced the programmed cell death (Messmer et al., 1996).

2.7. NO and Apoptosis

NO has been reported as both an anti-apoptotic and a proapoptotic molecule. During physiological conditions NO act as anti-apoptotic molecules however, most of the research reports have suggested it as pro-apoptotic molecule which depends on its cellular concentration and successive reaction of this free radical with other metals or reactive species. NO could directly bound to cytochrome-c oxidase and induces the formation of superoxide in mitochondria which further generate the $ONOO^-$. Such generated $ONOO^-$ inhibits the mitochondrial complex I, II, III and IV in either reversible or irreversible manner (Ghasemi et al., 2018; Stewart et al., 2002). Concentration dependent effect of NO has also been reported on the mitochondrial permeability and apoptosis (Lin et al., 1995; Brookes et al., 2000). $ONOO^-$ also affect the mitochondrial membrane integrity thus transient permeability, cytochrome–c release, mitochondrial antioxidative enzyme like SOD, mitochondrial DNA and causes mitochondrial swelling (Brown, 1999; Pearce et al., 2004, Folkes et al. 2014). Such varied adverse effect of NO is beneficial to cancerous cells and being utilized in exploration of cell specific anticancer therapies (Messmer et al., 1994) however, in neurodegenerative disease such adverse effects of NO are considered to be as pathogenic. Moreover, NO-induced apoptosis is related to the increase in the Bax/Bcl-2 ratio, which in turn leads to increase in mitochondrial permeability and cytochrome c release and caspases activation (Kolb, 2000). Various signaling factors like JNK/SAPK, p38 MAPK, c-jun/c-fos and various other proapoptotic factors migrate and initiate the apoptotic signaling in oxidative stress mediated damage (Kang and Chae, 2003; Verheij et al., 1996). However, controversial reports indicating the anti-apoptotic effects of NO mediated through death receptors as well as mediated through mitochondrion has also been suggested. Reports have showed that the S-nitrosylation capability of NO modify the proteins related to apoptosis including inhibition of caspase 3 (Saligrama et al., 2014), caspase 1 (Kim et al., 1998) and caspase 9 and the release of Bax (Thippeswamy et al., 2001). At physiological level NO inhibits the mitochondrial permeability transition pore (MPTP) formation and cytochrome c release (Brookes et al., 2000) thus offer antiapoptotic effects. NO also induces the expression of genes including HSP70 (Xu et al., 1997) that inhibits the Apaf-1 oligomerization by binding to its caspase domain (CARD) thus inhibits the formation of apoptosome (Beere et al., 2000). NO mediated direct inhibition of cytochrome c release has also been reported through activation of HSP70 (Mosser et al., 1997). NO could also regulate the level of antiapoptotic protein Bcl-2 involving guanylate cyclase activation and inhibition of Bcl-2 (Genaro et al., 1995; Kim et al., 1997). In neuronal PC12 cells and U937 immune cells, the anti-apoptotic effects of NO are linked to cGMP production, which suppresses cytochrome c release and ceramide generation (Fiscus, 2002). Both NO and cGMP offered protection to lymphocytes from apoptosis by maintaining Bcl-2 levels through the activation of Akt/PKB and inhibition of the pro-apoptotic Bad and procaspase-9 (Genaro et al., 1995). NO also exert the cGMP independent cytoprotective pathway as observed in endothelial cells (Kwon et al., 2001).

2.8. NO and Autophagy

Autophagy is an intracellular bulk degradation process that is required for the removal of protein aggregates and damaged organelles to prevent their adverse effects on physiological processes including immunity, development as well as pathological mechanisms involved in cancer and neurodegenerative diseases (Mizushima et al., 2008). Autophagy initiates with the formation of phagophores that elongate and engulf a portion of the cytoplasm to form mature autophagosomes which fuse with lysosomes to form autolysosomes, containing acidic lysosomal hydrolases to degrade the engulfed contents. This is tightly regulated pathway which stimulated during cellular stress, hypoxia, protein aggregation, DNA damage, ROS generation, damaged organelles or in presence of any pathogens. Role of NO and other RNS on autophagy have been investigated in last decade due to its ubiquitous expression in the cardiovascular, nervous, and immune systems and capability of eliciting a multitude of physiological responses, such as blood flow regulation and tissue responses to hypoxia (Foster et al., 2009). In murine cardiac HL-1 cells LPS induced autophagy has been observed which is mediated by increased level of endogenous NO and could be attenuated by NOS inhibitor N(G)-nitro-L-arginine methyl ester (L-NAME) (Huan et al., 2009). ONOO⁻ mediated increased protein tyrosine nitration is also associated with autophagy-lysosome activation as observed in cultured endothelial cells involving role of LC3II/I, GFP-LC3 puncta accumulation, lamp2 and cathepsin B activation (Fetterman et al., 2016). Augmented level of NO could also nityrosylate the PTEN, a tumor suppressor gene (Numajiri et al., 2011) and also the regulator of Akt/mTOR pathway thus inhibits the autophagy and promotes the cell viability (He et al., 2009). This NO mediated nitrosylation of PTEN is reported to be useful in cancerous cells/xenograft tumors with use of NOS inhibitor L-NAME however, its direct association in neuronal physiology and pathology remain to be elucidated. In neurons S-nitrosylation of PTEN leads to its degradation through ubiquitin ligase NEDD4-1 involving ubiquitin and Akt cascade (Kwak et al., 2010). Autophagy is also associated with ER stress related factors like Grp78/BiP which is considered as an obligatory factor for autophagy and may function at the phagophore expansion (Wang et al., 2015). Other ER stressors like tunicamycin is also reported to cause autophagic cell death as observed in kidney tubular cells (Kawakami et al., 2009). NO could also nitrosylate the other signaling factors like JNK1 and IKKβ (inhibitor of nuclear factor kappa-B kinase) to reduce their activity and Bcl-2 phosphorylation which further activates the mTORC1 (mammalian target of rapamycin complex 1), IKKβ- and TSC2-dependent manner (Sarkar et al., 2011). However, one controversial report suggested that reduced NO synthesis induces autophagy and protects against neurodegeneration in models of Huntington's disease (Browne and Beal,

2006). It has also been reported that disruption of autophagosome-lysosome fusion by bafilomycin A inhibited eNOS activation, suggesting involvement of autophagy in maintaining NO bioavailability (Fetterman et al., 2016) demonstrating their correlation however, lacunae remain to be filled with in depth studies.

2.9. NO and Glial Cells

Both astrocytes and microglial cells are the majorly populated glial cells of the brain which supports various physiological functions of neurons. Astrocytes are known to play critical role in various neural processes such as sleep, breathing coordination, learning and memory, maintain the blood-brain barrier, ion homeostasis, regulates oxidative stress and control the synaptic function including synaptophysin and pruning (Lundgaard et al., 2014; Wang et al., 2015). Astrocytes interact with neurons through astrocytic projections, enables astrocytic-neuron cross-talk to protect the neurons against cellular damage and prevent various neurodegenerative signaling (Rizor et al., 2019). nNOS expressed in astrocytes, synaptic spines and near the blood-brain barrier within CNS (Yuste et al., 2015). Both astrocytes and microglial cells of the brain express iNOS abundantly which has physiological functions and overexpressed during pathological conditions (Saha and Pahan, 2006; Singh, 2020). Reports have suggested that exposure of environmental toxins such as rotenone, paraquat, MPTP (1-methyl-4-phenyl-1,2,3,6-tetrahydropyridine) to astrocytes prompt these to express iNOS and increase the level of NO leading to astrocytes activation mediated generation of nitrosative and oxidative environment in brain (Booth et al., 2017). Astrocyte play physiological role in neuronal maintenance as these provides glutamine to neurons which transforms into glutamate for neurotransmission. Glial cells mediated augmented inflammatory responses as reviewed previously (Singh et al., 2011) further increased the iNOS and nNOS expression and contribute to reactive astrogliosis which release NO into extracellular space and is taken up by neuron, directing the neuronal cells towards depleted activity of antioxidant machinery, increased lipid peroxidation, DNA damage, and mitochondrial dysfunction which collectively caused neuronal death (Teismann and Schulz, 2004). Cytokine release through NO overproduction consequently produced high levels of ONOO⁻ which inhibited the mitochondrial complex I, II, III and IV activity and cause mitochondrial dysfunction in the rat primary astrocyte-neuronal co-culture, a process which was reversed after removal of reactive astrocyte (Stewert et al., 2002). Pathological conditions related activated astrocytes mediated increased expression of iNOS thus NO facilitate the NFkB mediated activation of caspases to execute the neuronal death (Singh, 2020; Swanson et al., 2004). Simultaneously, NO mediated S-nitrosylation of NFkB hindered its binding capacity to DNA, therefore obstructing transcriptional activation of various genes (Singh et al., 2020) and further investigation is required to establish their functional association. Till now we have discussed the diverse role of NO in consociation with various organelles and signaling while in the following sections we will be providing the available evidences in context to role of NO in CNS-neurodegenerative diseases.

3. EVIDENCES FOR ROLE OF NO IN CNS-NEURODEGENERATIVE DISEASES

3.1. Evidences for Role of NO in AD Pathology

Alzheimer's disease is progressive neurodegenerative disorder mainly characterized by specific loss of synapse and cholinergic neurons responsible for cognitive responses. Pathological markers of AD are intracellular deposition of neurofibrillary tangles formed due to hyperphosphorylation of tau protein and extracellular deposition of amyloid beta plaques (Liu and L., 2019). Kummer et al., (2011) reported that treatment of iNOS inhibitor to transgenic model of AD that is APP/PS1 mice exhibited the decreased expression of Aβ and cognitive dysfunction by limiting tyrosine nitrosylation of Aβ. It has also been reported that AD pathology related augmented expression of iNOS in glial cells and their activation mediated inflammatory and immune responses further contribute in NO and its metabolite induced neuronal death (Contestabile et al., 2012). AD pathology is very well associated with impairment of protein aggregation and degradation related mechanisms which also involve the NO mediated S-nitrosylation of proteins and their consequent misfolding and aggregation which further contribute in ER stress related death mechanisms (Wang et al., 2020; Uddin et al., 2020). Report by Honjo et al., (2014) demonstrated that S-nitrosylated ER chaperon PDI facilitate the tau related formation of neurofibrillary tangles (NFTs). NO also plays an important role in learning and memory, as it participates in NO/cGMP and CAM kinase II signaling of memory in hippocampus (Hossein et al., 2012). Controversially the neuroprotective role of eNOS has been reported in AD pathology. It has been shown that loss of eNOS led to increased expression of APP and BACE1 protein and Aβ level in brain (Austin et al., 2010, 2012).

3.2. Evidences for Role of NO in PD Pathology

Parkinson's disease is the second most common motor neurodegenerative disease characterized by tremor, postural rigidity, bradykinesia (Tiwari and Singh, 2020). These symptoms occur due to the loss of dopaminergic neurons in the substantia nigra pars compacta (SNpC) region of the brain (Tiwari and Singh, 2019) and biochemical features include the aggregation of PD related protein such as α-synuclein, chaperones and ubiquitin residues in the SNpC to form lewy body and lewy neurites (Picon-pages et al., 2019). High levels of NO and peroxynitrite have been reported in the serum of PD patients with a positive correlation between the NO surge and UPDRS scores (Kouti et al., 2013). Resistance to PD related pathology was observed in iNOS deficient mice administered with MPTP (Liberatore et al., 1999). Similarly, iNOS inhibitor 7-nitroindazol administration in rats mitigated the rotenone induced neurotoxicity and occurrence of PD like symptoms (He et al., 2003). Previously we have also reported the role of NO in generating nitrosative and oxidative stress, activating proinflammatory pathways, mitochondrial dysfunction as well as ER stress and proteosome impairment during disease (Singh and Dikshit, 2007; Goswami et al., 2014; Gupta et al., 2019). The nitration of α-synuclein through tyrosine residue has been reported in the brain of PD patients which further promotes the aggregation of α-synuclein, hindering its binding to the neurotransmitter vesicles and lead to the neurotoxicity (Burai et al., 2015; Duda et al., 2000). Rate limiting enzyme of dopamine synthesis tyrosine hydroxylase could also be nitrotyrosylated by NO thus impairs its activity thereby halting the dopamine synthesis and initiating PD pathogenesis (Ara et al., 1998; Ekhteiari et al., 2018). NO reacts with superoxide to generate the peroxynitrite which inhibits the dopamine transporter function preventing its uptake from synaptic cleft and hence the related physiological signaling (Park et al., 2002). Parkin is S-nitrosylated during PD which not only impedes mitophagy and proteasomal degradation of misfolded proteins, but also leads to aggregation and accumulation of various Parkin substrates such as synphilin-1 promulgating the disease progression (Chung et al., 2004). NO contributes to PD pathology due to its role in several signaling pathways and reducing NO levels may lead to amelioration of PD pathogenesis and disease related neuronal death however concentration-based studies are needed in this direction*.

3.3. Evidences for Role of NO in HD Pathology

Huntington's disease is a neurodegenerative disease producing dementia and involuntary movements characterized by neuronal loss in the striatum (Vonsattel et al., 1985). It is an autosomal dominant disease caused by an expansion of a CAG trinucleotide repeat on the huntingtin (htt) gene located on the short arm of chromosome 4. Most HD patients have CAG repeat sequences that vary from 40 to 49 repeats and they develop symptoms between the third and the fifth decades of their life (Lucotte et al., 1995). In HD, htt has an expanded polyglutamine tract at the extreme N-terminus, which triggers neurotoxicity through several proposed mechanisms involving excitotoxicity by NMDA receptors (Zeron et al., 2004), impairment in vesicle trafficking, lack of neurotrophins and transcriptional effects (Ross, 2004). There are two putative pathways have been suggested which link HD with NO production involving htt/HAP-1 (htt-associated protein)/calmodulin/NOS and CREB binding protein (CBP) /htt/NOS. HAP-1 forms a complex with htt which could bind to calmodulin, the main regulator of nNOS and eNOS (Li et al., 1995; Bao et al., 1996). When htt/HAP-1 complex is mutated, its affinity for calmodulin increases, preventing nNOS activation (Bao et al., 1996). On the other hand, it has also been found that Ca^{2+} regulates the nNOS expression through a promoter located on exon 2 of the nNOS gene (Sasaki et al., 2000). This promoter responds to CBP which binds to two critical cAMP/Ca^{2+} response elements, which are immediately upstream of the nNOS transcription start site. It has been found that htt interacts with CBP and represses nNOS transcription (Sasaki et al., 2000; Steffan et al., 2000). Moreover, CREB/CBP complex is under the control of the calmodulin kinases (Chawla et al., 1998), which could be inactive due to the interaction of htt/HAP-1 with calmodulin. Both in experimental models of HD as well as in brain of HD patients the increased level of NO has been reported suggesting its pathological role in disease onset (Butterfield et al., 2001; Chen et al., 2000).

3.4. Evidences for Role of NO in ALS Pathology

Amyotrophic lateral sclerosis (ALS) is a devastating neurodegenerative disease characterized by progressive loss of motor neurons in motor cortex, brain stem and spinal cord that results in muscle weakness, paralysis and ultimately to death. There are nearly 30 gene involved in the ALS pathogenesis, in which SOD1 was the first gene to be identified as involved in ALS (Rosen et al., 1993). ALS pathology is related to the mutations in gene for copper/zinc SOD1. The main function of the SOD1enzyme is to protect the tissue from the oxidative stress by dismutating the superoxide radicals ($O_2^{\cdot -}$) into the molecular oxygen (O_2) and less reactive hydrogen peroxides (H_2O_2) (Pansarasa et al., 2018). During the physiological conditions the increased level of superoxide is controlled by its scavenging through SOD however, the mutation of SOD lead to increased level of superoxide which further reacts with NO to form the more toxic ONOO⁻ thus worsen the diseased conditions and cause the neuronal death. Deprivation of neurotrophic factor is also one of the pathological reason for neuronal death. It has been reported that BDNF deprived motor neurons exhibit the increased expression of nNOS and consociated activation of FasL-FADD pathway leading to activation of apoptotic (Estevez et al., 1998). In the neuronal cells, peroxynitrite reacts with SOD to form nitronium like intermediates, that nitrates tyrosine residues in the neurofilaments and form nitrotyrosine that effects drastically in protein structure and functions to modulates synaptic plasticity (Beckman et al., 1993; Valle et al., 2017). It is also reported that increased NO production due to the up regulation of NOS, activates the glial cells to release cytokines that causes inflammatory response followed by motor neuronal cell death during ALS (Giorgio et al., 2008).

FUTURE PERSPECTIVE AND CONCLUSION

Research in last two-three decades has suggested the considerable role of NO in pathogenesis of neurodegenerative diseases. In this chapter we have discussed about the major involvement of NO in various neurodegenerative signaling pathways. Findings suggested that NO has both direct and indirect involvement in neuronal death primarily through energy crisis as it affects the mitochondrion functionality. However, it affects various other physiological mechanisms which should also be considered during development of therapeutics of discussed neurodegenerative diseases. Studies are available indicating the protective effect of NOS inhibitors however the broad and multi-aspect studies are needed as NO plays significant role in cellular physiology. This chapters gives the overview of role of NO in neurodegeneration and how this information could be implied in development of disease therapeutics.

REFERENCES

Ahmad, R., Hussain, A., & Ahsan, H. (2019). Peroxynitrite: cellular pathology and implications in autoimmunity. *Journal of Immunoassay and Immunochemistry*, 1–16. doi:10.1080/15321819.2019.1583109.

Ara, J., Przedborski, S., Naini, A. B., Jackson-Lewis, V., Trifiletti, R. R., Horwitz, J., & Ischiropoulos, H. (1998). Inactivation of tyrosine hydroxylase by nitration following exposure to peroxynitrite and 1-methyl-4-phenyl-1,2,3,6-tetrahydropyridine (MPTP). *Proceedings of the National Academy of Sciences*, 95(13), 7659–7663. doi:10.1073/pnas.95.13.7659.

Asano, S., Fukuda, Y., Beck, F., Aufderheide, A., Forster, F., Danev, R., & Baumeister, W. (2015). A molecular census of 26S proteasomes in intact neurons. *Science*, 347(6220), 439–442. doi:10.1126/science.1261197.

Austin S. A., d'Uscio L. V. and Katusic Z. S. (2012) Supplementation of nitric oxide attenuates AbetaPP and BACE1 protein in cerebral microcirculation of eNOS-deficient mice. *J. Alzheimers Dis.* 33, 29–33.

Austin S. A., Santhanam A. V. and Katusic Z. S. (2010) Endothelial nitric oxide modulates expression and processing of amyloid precursor protein. *Circ. Res.* 107, 1498–1502.

Baillet, A.; Chanteperdrix, V.; Trocme, C.; Casez, P.; Garrel, C.; & Besson, G. The role of oxidative stress in amyotrophic lateral sclerosis and Parkinson's disease. *Neurochem. Res.* 2010, 35, 1530–1537.

Bal, N., Roshchin, M., Salozhin, S., & Balaban, P. (2016). Nitric Oxide Upregulates Proteasomal Protein Degradation in Neurons. *Cellular and Molecular Neurobiology*, 37(5), 763–769. doi:10.1007/s10571-016-0413-9.

Bao, J., Sharp, A. H., Wagster, M. V., Becher, M., Schilling, G., Ross, C. A., Dawson, V. L., Dawson, T. M., 1996. Expansion of polyglutamine repeatin huntingtin leads to abnormal protein interactions involving calmodulin. *Proc. Natl. Acad. Sci. USA.* 93, 5037–5042.

Beal MF. Excitotoxicity and nitric oxide in Parkinson's disease pathogenesis. *Ann Neurol.* 1998;44(3 Suppl 1):S110-S114. doi:10.1002/ana.410440716.

Beal, M. F. Excitotoxicity and nitric oxide in Parkinson's disease pathogenesis. *Ann. Neurol.* 1998, 44 (Suppl. 1), S110–S114.

Beckman JS, Carson M, Smith CD, Koppenol WH. ALS, SOD and peroxynitrite. *Nature.* 1993;364(6438):584. doi:10.1038/364584a0

Beere, H. M., Wolf, B. B., Cain, K., Mosser, D. D., Mahboubi, A., Kuwana, T., Green, D. R. (2000). Heat-shock protein 70 inhibits apoptosis by preventing recruitment of procaspase-9 to the Apaf-1 apoptosome. *Nature Cell Biology*, 2(8), 469–475. doi:10.1038/35019501.

Biswas, J., Gupta, S., Verma, D. K., Gupta, P., Singh, A., Tiwari, S., Singh, S. (2018). Involvement of glucose related energy crisis and endoplasmic reticulum stress: Insinuation of streptozotocin induced Alzheimer's like pathology. *Cellular Signalling*, 42, 211–226. doi:10.1016/j.cellsig.2017.10.018.

Booth, H. D. E.; Hirst, W. D.; Wade-Martins, R. The Role of Astrocyte Dysfunction in Parkinson's Disease Pathogenesis. *Trends Neurosci.* 2017, 40:358–370.

Bradley, S. A., & Steinert, J. R. (2016). Nitric Oxide-Mediated Posttranslational Modifications: Impacts at the Synapse. *Oxidative Medicine and Cellular Longevity*, 2016, 1–9. doi:10.1155/2016/5681036.

Brookes, P. S., Salinas, E. P., Darley-Usmar, K., Eiserich, J. P., Freeman, B. A., Darley-Usmar, V. M., & Anderson, P. G. (2000). Concentration-dependent Effects of Nitric Oxide on Mitochondrial Permeability Transition and CytochromecRelease. *Journal of Biological Chemistry*, 275(27), 20474–20479. doi:10.1074/jbc.m001077200.

Brown GC. Nitric oxide and mitochondrial respiration. *Biochim Biophys Acta.* 1999;1411(2-3):351-369. doi:10.1016/s0005-2728(99)00025-0.

Brown, G. C. (1999). Nitric oxide and mitochondrial respiration. Biochimica et Biophysica Acta (BBA) - *Bioenergetics*, 1411(2-3), 351–369. doi:10.1016/s0005-2728(99)00025-0.

Browne, S. E., & Beal, M. F. (2006). Oxidative Damage in Huntington's Disease Pathogenesis. *Antioxidants & Redox Signaling*, 8(11-12), 2061–2073. doi:10.1089/ars.2006.8.2061

Burai, R., Ait-Bouziad, N., Chiki, A., & Lashuel, H. A. (2015). Elucidating the Role of Site-Specific Nitration of α-Synuclein in the Pathogenesis of Parkinson's Disease via Protein Semisynthesis and Mutagenesis. *Journal of the American Chemical Society*, 137(15), 5041–5052. doi:10.1021/ja5131726.

Butterfield, D. A., Howard, B. J., LaFontaine, M. A., 2001. Brain oxidativestress in animal models of accelerated aging and the age-relatedneurodegenerative disorders: Alzheimer's disease and Huntington'sdisease. *Curr. Med. Chem.* 8, 815–828.

Cenini, G., Lloret, A., & Cascella, R. (2019). Oxidative Stress in Neurodegenerative Diseases: From a Mitochondrial Point of View. *Oxidative Medicine and Cellular Longevity,* 2019, 1–18. doi:10.1155/2019/2105607

Chawla, S., Hardingham, G. E., Quinn, D. R., Bading, H., 1998. CBP: asignal-regulated transcriptional coactivator controlled by nuclear calciumand CaM kinase IV. *Science* 281, 1505–1509.

Chen, C.-F., Wang, D., Hwang, C. P., Liu, H. W., Wei, J., Lee, R. P., & Chen, H. I. (2001). The Protective Effect of Niacinamide on Ischemia-Reperfusion-Induced Liver Injury. *Journal of Biomedical Science,* 8(6), 446–452. doi:10.1159/000046165.

Chen, M., Ona, V. O., Li, M., Ferrante, R. J., Fink, K. B., Zhu, S., Bian, J., Guo, L., Farrell, L. A., Hersch, S. M., Hobbs, W., Vonsattel, J. P., Cha, J. H., Friedlander, R. M., 2000. Minocycline inhibits caspase-1 andcaspase-3 expression and delays mortality in a transgenic mouse modelof Huntington disease. *Nat. Med.* 6, 797–801.

Cho DH, Nakamura T, Fang J, Cieplak P, Godzik A, Gu Z, and Lipton SA. S-Nitrosylation of Drp1 mediates β-amyloid-related mitochondrial fission and neuronal injury. *Science* 324: 102-105, 2009.

Chu Q, Martinez TF, Novak SW, Donaldson CJ, Tan D, Vaughan JM, Chang T, Diedrich JK, Andrade L, Kim A, Zhang T, Manor U, Saghatelian A. Regulation of the ER stress response by a mitochondrial microprotein. *Nat Commun.* 2019 Oct 25;10(1):4883. doi: 10.1038/s41467-019-12816-z. PMID: 31653868; PMCID: PMC6814811.

Chung K. K., Thomas B., Li X., Pletnikova O., Troncoso J. C., Marsh L., Dawson V. L., and Dawson T. M. S-Nitrosylation of parkin regulates ubiquitination and compromises parkin's protective function. *Science* 304: 1328-1331, 2004.

Contestabile, A., Monti, B., & Polazzi, E. (2012). Neuronal-glial Interactions Define the Role of Nitric Oxide in Neural Functional Processes. *Current Neuropharmacology,* 10(4), 303–310. doi:10.2174/157015912804499465

Di Giorgio, F. P., Boulting, G. L., Bobrowicz, S., & Eggan, K. C. (2008). Human Embryonic Stem Cell-Derived Motor Neurons Are Sensitive to the Toxic Effect of Glial Cells Carrying an ALS-Causing Mutation. *Cell Stem Cell*, 3(6), 637–648. doi:10.1016/j.stem.2008.09.017

Doble A. The role of excitotoxicity in neurodegenerative disease: implications for therapy. *Pharmacol Ther.* 1999;81(3):163-221. doi:10.1016/s0163-7258(98)00042-4.

Dong X. X., Wang Y., Qin Z. H. Molecular mechanisms of excitotoxicity and their relevance to pathogenesis of neurodegenerative diseases. *Acta Pharmacol Sin.* 2009;30(4):379-387. doi:10.1038/aps.2009.24.

Doulias P. T., Tenopoulou M., Greene J. L., Raju K., and Ischiropoulos H. Nitric oxide regulates mitochondrial fatty acid metabolism through reversible protein S-nitrosylation. *Sci. Signal.* 6: rs1, 2013.

Duda, J. E., Giasson, B. I., Chen, Q., Gur, T. L., Hurtig, H. I., Stern, M. B., Trojanowski, J. Q. (2000). Widespread Nitration of Pathological Inclusions in Neurodegenerative Synucleinopathies. *The American Journal of Pathology*, 157(5), 1439–1445. doi:10.1016/s0002-9440(10)64781-5.

Ekhteiari Salmas R., Durdagi S., Gulhan M. F., Duruyurek M., Abdullah H. I., Selamoglu Z. The effects of pollen, propolis, and caffeic acid phenethyl ester on tyrosine hydroxylase activity and total RNA levels in hypertensive rats caused by nitric oxide synthase inhibition: experimental, docking and molecular dynamic studies. *J Biomol Struct*

Dyn. 2018 Feb;36(3):609-620. doi: 10.1080/07391102.2017.1288660. Epub 2017 Feb 15. PMID: 28132600.

Estévez, A. G., Spear, N., Manuel, S. M., Radi, R., Henderson, C. E., Barbeito, L., & Beckman, J. S. (1998). Nitric Oxide and Superoxide Contribute to Motor Neuron Apoptosis Induced by Trophic Factor Deprivation. *The Journal of Neuroscience*, 18(3), 923–931. doi:10.1523/jneurosci.18-03-00923.1998.

Fetterman, J. L., Holbrook, M., Flint, N., Feng, B., Bretón-Romero, R., Linder, E. A., Vita, J. A. (2016). Restoration of autophagy in endothelial cells from patients with diabetes mellitus improves nitric oxide signaling. *Atherosclerosis,* 247, 207–217. doi:10.1016/j.atherosclerosis.2016.01.043.

Fiscus, R. R., 2002. Involvement of cyclic GMP and protein kinase G in theregulation of apoptosis and survival in neural cells. *Neurosignals* 11,175–190.

Foster, G. E., Brugniaux, J. V., Pialoux, V., Duggan, C. T. C., Hanly, P. J., Ahmed, S. B., & Poulin, M. J. (2009). Cardiovascular and cerebrovascular responses to acute hypoxia following exposure to intermittent hypoxia in healthy humans. *The Journal of Physiology*, 587(13), 3287–3299. doi:10.1113/jphysiol.2009.171553

Genaro A. M., Hortelano S., Alvarez A., Martínez C., Boscá L. Splenic B lymphocyte programmed cell death is prevented by nitric oxide release through mechanisms involving sustained Bcl-2 levels. *J Clin Invest.* 1995;95(4):1884-1890. doi:10.1172/JCI117869.

Ghasemi, M., Mayasi, Y., Hannoun, A., Eslami, S. M., & Carandang, R. (2018). Nitric Oxide and Mitochondrial Function in Neurological Diseases. *Neuroscience,* 376, 48–71. doi:10.1016/j.neuroscience.2018.02.017.

Ghemrawi R., Khair M. Endoplasmic Reticulum Stress and Unfolded Protein Response in Neurodegenerative Diseases. *Int J Mol Sci.* 2020 Aug 25;21(17):E6127. doi: 10.3390/ijms21176127. PMID: 32854418.

Giasson B. I., Duda J. E., Murray I. V., Chen Q., Souza J. M., Hurtig H. I., Ischiropoulos H., Trojanowski J. Q., and Lee V. M. Oxidative damage linked to neurodegeneration by selective alpha-synuclein nitration in synucleinopathy lesions. *Science* 290: 985-989, 2000.

Goswami, P., Gupta, S., Biswas, J., Joshi, N., Swarnkar, S., Nath, C., & Singh, S. (2014). Endoplasmic Reticulum Stress Plays a Key Role in Rotenone-Induced Apoptotic Death of Neurons. *Molecular Neurobiology, 53*(1), 285–298. doi:10.1007/s12035-014-9001-5

Gupta S., Mishra K. P., Kumar B., Singh S. B., Ganju L. Andrographolide Mitigates Unfolded Protein Response Pathway andApoptosis Involved in Chikungunya virus *Infection* (2020). doi:10.2174/1386207323999200818165029.

Gupta, S., Biswas, J., Gupta, P., Singh, A., Tiwari, S., Mishra, A., & Singh, S. (2019). Salubrinal attenuates nitric oxide mediated PERK:IRE1α: ATF-6 signaling and DNA damage in neuronal cells. *Neurochemistry International,* 104581. doi:10.1016/j.neuint.2019.104581

Han J. Y., Kang M. J., Kim K. H., Han P. L., Kim H. S., Ha J. Y., and Son J. H. Nitric oxide induction of Parkin translocation in PTEN-induced putative kinase 1 (PINK1) deficiency: functional role of neuronal nitric oxide synthase during mitophagy. *J Biol Chem* 290: 10325-10335, 2015.

Hardy, M.; Zielonka, J.; Karoui, H.; Sikora, A.; Michalski, R.; Podsiadly, R.; Lopez, M.; Vasquez-Vivar, J.; Kalyanaraman, B.; & Ouari, O. Detection and Characterization of Reactive Oxygen and Nitrogen Species in Biological Systems by Monitoring Species-Specific Products. Antioxid. *Redox Signal.* 2018, 28, 1416–1432.

Hashemy S. I., Johansson C., Berndt C., Lillig C. H., Holmgren A. (2007) Oxidation and S-nitrosylation of cysteines in human cytosolic and mitochondrial glutaredoxins: effects on structure and activity. *J Biol Chem* 282:14428-14436.

He, C., & Klionsky, D. J. (2009). Regulation Mechanisms and Signaling Pathways of Autophagy. *Annual Review of Genetics*, 43(1), 67–93. doi:10.1146/annurev-genet-102808-114910

He, Y., Imam, S. Z., Dong, Z., Jankovic, J., Ali, S. F., Appel, S. H., & Le, W. (2003). Role of nitric oxide in rotenone-induced nigro-striatal injury. *Journal of Neurochemistry,* 86(6), 1338–1345. doi:10.1046/j.1471-4159.2003.01938.x

Honjo, Y., Horibe, T., Torisawa, A., Ito, H., Nakanishi, A., Mori, H., Kawakami, K. (2013). Protein Disulfide Isomerase P5-Immunopositive Inclusions in Patients with Alzheimer's Disease. *Journal of Alzheimer's Disease*, 38(3), 601–609. doi:10.3233/jad-130632.

Hosseini M., Pourganji M., Khodabandehloo F., Soukhtanloo M., Zabihi H. (2012) Protective Eject of L-Arginine against Oxidative Damage as a Possible Mechanism of its Beneficial Properties on Spatial Learning in Ovariectomized Rats. *Basic Clinical Neurosci* 3: 36-44.

Kang, Y. J., & Chae, S. W. (2003). JNK/SAPK is required in nitric oxide-induced apoptosis in osteoblasts. *Archives of Pharmacal Research*, 26(11), 937–942. doi:10.1007/bf02980203

Kawakami, T., Inagi, R., Takano, H., Sato, S., Ingelfinger, J. R., Fujita, T., & Nangaku, M. (2009). Endoplasmic reticulum stress induces autophagy in renal proximal tubular cells. *Nephrology Dialysis Transplantation*, 24(9), 2665–2672. doi:10.1093/ndt/gfp215.

Kim Y. M., Talanian R. V., Li J., Billiar T. R. Nitric oxide prevents IL-1beta and IFN-gamma-inducing factor (IL-18) release from macrophages by inhibiting caspase-1 (IL-1beta-converting enzyme). *J Immunol.* 1998;161(8):4122-4128.

Kim, W. K., Choi, Y. B., Rayudu, P. V., Das, P., Asaad, W., Arnelle, D. R., Lipton, S. A. (1999). Attenuation of NMDA Receptor Activity and Neurotoxicity by Nitroxyl Anion, NO−. *Neuron*, 24(2), 461–469. doi:10.1016/s0896-6273(00)80859-4.

Kim, Y. M., Talanian, R. V., Billiar, T. R., 1997. Nitric oxide inhibits apoptosisby preventing increases in caspase-3-like activity via two distinctmechanisms. *J. Biol. Chem.* 272, 31138–31148.

Kolb, J. P. (2000). Mechanisms involved in the pro- and anti-apoptotic role of NO in human leukemia. *Leukemia*, 14(9), 1685–1694. doi:10.1038/sj.leu.2401896.

Kolodziejski, P. J., Musial, A., Koo, J. S., & Eissa, N. T. (2002). Ubiquitination of inducible nitric oxide synthase is required for its degradation. *Proceedings of the National Academy of Sciences*, 99(19), 12315–12320. doi:10.1073/pnas.192345199.

Kouti L., Noroozian M., Akhondzadeh S., et al. Nitric oxide and peroxynitrite serum levels in Parkinson's disease: correlation of oxidative stress and the severity of the disease. *European Review for Medical and Pharmacological Sciences.* 2013 Apr;17(7):964-970.

Kummer M. P., Hermes M., Delekarte A., et al. Nitration of tyrosine 10 critically enhances amyloid β aggregation and plaque formation. *Neuron.* 2011;71(5):833-844. doi:10.1016/j.neuron.2011.07.001.

Kummer M. P., Hermes M., Delekarte A., Hammerschmidt T., Kumar S., Terwel D., Walter J., Pape H. C., Konig S., Roeber S., Jessen F., Klockgether T, Korte M, and Heneka MT. Nitration of tyrosine 10 critically enhances amyloid beta aggregation and plaque formation. *Neuron* 71: 833-844, 2011.

Kwak, Y. D., Ma, T., Diao, S., Zhang, X., Chen, Y., Hsu, J., Liao, F. F. (2010). NO signaling and S-nitrosylation regulate PTEN inhibition in neurodegeneration. *Molecular Neurodegeneration,* 5(1), 49. doi:10.1186/1750-1326-5-49.

Kwon, Y. G., Min, J. K., Kim, K. M., Lee, D. J., Billiar, T. R., Kim, Y. M., 2001.Sphingosine 1-phosphate protects human umbilical vein endothelialcells from serum-deprived apoptosis by nitric oxide production. *J. Biol. Chem.* 276, 10627–10633.

Lau A., Tymianski M. Glutamate receptors, neurotoxicity and neurodegeneration. *Pflugers Arch.* 2010;460(2):525-542. doi:10.1007/s00424-010-0809-1.

Li, X. J., Li, S. H., Sharp, A. H., Nucifora Jr., F. C., Schilling, G., Lanahan, A.,Worley, P., Snyder, S. H., Ross, C. A., 1995. A huntingtin-associatedprotein enriched in brain with implications for pathology. Nature 378,398–402.

Liberatore, G. T., Jackson-Lewis, V., Vukosavic, S., Mandir, A. S., Vila, M., McAuliffe, W. G., Przedborski, S. (1999). Inducible nitric oxide synthase stimulates dopaminergic neurodegeneration in the MPTP model of Parkinson disease. *Nature Medicine*, 5(12), 1403–1409. doi:10.1038/70978 .

Lin, C. (1995). Dimethyl Sulfoxide Suppresses Apoptosis in Burkitt's Lymphoma Cells. *Experimental Cell Research*, 216(2), 403–410. doi:10.1006/excr.1995.1051.

Liu J. and Li L. (2019) Targeting Autophagy for the Treatment of Alzheimer's Disease: Challenges and Opportunities. *Front. Mol. Neurosci.* 12:203. doi: 10.3389/fnmol.2019.00203

Loeb, L. A., & Preston, B. D. (1986). Mutagenesis by Apurinic/Apyrimidinic Sites. *Annual Review of Genetics*, 20(1), 201–230. doi:10.1146/annurev.ge.20.120186.001221.

Lucotte, G., Turpin, J. C., Riess, O., Epplen, J. T., Siedlaczk, I., Loirat, F.,Hazout, S., 1995. Confidence intervals for predicted age of onset, giventhe size of (CAG)n repeat, in Huntington's disease. *Hum. Genet.* 95,231–232.

Lucotte, G., Turpin, J. C., Riess, O., Epplen, J. T., Siedlaczk, I., Loirat, F., Hazout, S., 1995. Confidence intervals for predicted age of onset, giventhe size of (CAG)n repeat, in Huntington's disease. *Hum. Genet.* 95,231–232.

Lundgaard, I., Osório, M. J., Kress, B. T., Sanggaard, S., & Nedergaard, M. (2014). White matter astrocytes in health and disease. *Neuroscience,* 276, 161–173. doi:10.1016/j.neuroscience.2013.10.050.

Luo, C., Gangadharan, V., Bali, K. K., Xie, R. G., Agarwal, N., Kurejova, M., Kuner, R. (2012). Presynaptically Localized Cyclic GMP-Dependent Protein Kinase 1 Is a Key Determinant of Spinal Synaptic Potentiation and Pain Hypersensitivity. *PLoS Biology,* 10(3), e1001283. doi:10.1371/journal.pbio.1001283.

Messmer, U. K., & BRÜNE, B. (1996). Nitric oxide-induced apoptosis: p53-dependent and p53-independent signalling pathways. *Biochemical Journal,* 319(1), 299–305. doi:10.1042/bj3190299.

Meßmer, U. K., Ankarcrona, M., Nicotera, P., & Brüne, B. (1994). P. 53 expression in nitric oxide-induced apoptosis. *FEBS Letters*, 355(1), 23–26. doi:10.1016/0014-5793(94)01161-3.

Mizushima, N., Levine, B., Cuervo, A. M., & Klionsky, D. J. (2008). Autophagy fights disease through cellular self-digestion. *Nature,* 451(7182), 1069–1075. doi:10.1038/nature06639.

Mosser, D. D., Caron, A. W., Bourget, L., Denis-Larose, C., & Massie, B. (1997). Role of the human heat shock protein hsp70 in protection against stress-induced apoptosis. *Molecular and Cellular Biology*, 17(9), 5317–5327. doi:10.1128/mcb.17.9.5317.

Musial, A., & Eissa, N. T. (2001). Inducible Nitric-oxide Synthase Is Regulated by the Proteasome Degradation Pathway. *Journal of Biological Chemistry*, 276(26), 24268–24273. doi:10.1074/jbc.m100725200.

Nakamura T., Wang L., Wong C. C., Scott F. L., Eckelman B. P., Han X., Tzitzilonis C., Meng F., Gu Z., Holland E. A., Clemente A. T., Okamoto S., Salvesen G. S., Riek R., Yates J. R., 3rd, and Lipton S. A. Transnitrosylation of XIAP regulates caspase-dependent neuronal cell death. *Mol. Cell* 39: 184-195, 2010.

Nakamura, T., & Lipton, S. A. (2019). Nitric Oxide-Dependent Protein Posttranslational Modifications Impair Mitochondrial Function and Metabolism to Contribute to Neurodegenerative Diseases. *Antioxidants & Redox Signaling*. doi:10.1089/ars.2019.7916.

Nakato, R., Ohkubo, Y., Konishi, A., Shibata, M., Kaneko, Y., Iwawaki, T., Uehara, T. (2015). Regulation of the unfolded protein response via S-nitrosylation of sensors of endoplasmic reticulum stress. *Scientific Reports*, 5, 14812. doi:10.1038/srep14812.

Nisoli E., Carruba M. O. Nitric oxide and mitochondrial biogenesis. *J Cell Sci.* 2006;119(Pt 14):2855-2862. doi:10.1242/jcs.03062

Nott, A., & Riccio, A. (2009). Nitric Oxide-mediated epigenetic mechanisms in developing neurons. *Cell Cycle*, 8(5), 725–730. doi:10.4161/cc.8.5.7805.

Numajiri N., Takasawa K., Nishiya T., et al. On-off system for PI3-kinase-Akt signaling through S-nitrosylation of phosphatase with sequence homology to tensin (PTEN). *Proc Natl Acad Sci USA.* 2011;108(25):10349-10354. doi:10.1073/pnas.1103503108.

Oh C. K., Sultan A., Platzer J., Dolatabadi N., Soldner F., McClatchy D. B., Diedrich J. K., Yates J. R., 3rd, Ambasudhan R., Nakamura T., Jaenisch R., and Lipton S. A. S-Nitrosylation of PINK1 Attenuates

PINK1/Parkin-Dependent Mitophagy in hiPSC-Based Parkinson's Disease Models. *Cell Rep* 21: 2171-2182, 2017.

Oyadomari S., Takeda K., Takiguchi M., Gotoh T., Matsumoto M., Wada I., Akira S., Araki E., Mori M. Nitric oxide-induced apoptosis in pancreatic β cells is mediated by the endoplasmic reticulum stress pathway. *Proc Natl Acad Sci USA*. 2001; 98: 10845–10850.

Oyadomari, S., Araki, E., & Mori, M. (2002). *APOPTOSIS,* 7(4), 335–345. doi:10.1023/a:1016175429877.

Pacher P., Beckman J. S., Liaudet L. Nitric oxide and peroxynitrite in health and disease. *Physiol Rev*. 2007;87(1):315-424. doi:10.1152/physrev.00029.2006.

Pansarasa, O., Bordoni, M., Diamanti, L., Sproviero, D., Gagliardi, S., & Cereda, C. (2018). SOD1 in Amyotrophic Lateral Sclerosis: "Ambivalent" Behavior Connected to the Disease. International *Journal of Molecular Sciences,* 19(5), 1345. doi:10.3390/ijms19051345.

Park, S. U., Ferrer, J. V., Javitch, J. A., & Kuhn, D. M. (2002). Peroxynitrite Inactivates the Human Dopamine Transporter by Modification of Cysteine 342: Potential Mechanism of Neurotoxicity in Dopamine Neurons. *The Journal of Neuroscience*, 22(11), 4399–4405. doi:10.1523/jneurosci.22-11-04399.2002.

Pearce, L. L., Kanai, A. J., Epperly, M. W., & Peterson, J. (2005). Nitrosative stress results in irreversible inhibition of purified mitochondrial complexes I and III without modification of cofactors. *Nitric Oxide*, 13(4), 254–263. doi:10.1016/j.niox.2005.07.010.

Picón-Pagès, P., Garcia-Buendia, J., & Muñoz, F. J. (2018). Functions and dysfunctions of nitric oxide in brain. Biochimica et Biophysica Acta (BBA) - *Molecular Basis of Disease*. doi:10.1016/j.bbadis.2018.11.007.

Pollard A. K., Craig E. L., Chakrabarti L. Mitochondrial Complex 1 Activity Measured by Spectrophotometry Is Reduced across All Brain Regions in Ageing and More Specifically in Neurodegeneration. *PLoS One*. 2016;11(6):e0157405. Published 2016 Jun 22. doi:10.1371/journal.pone.0157405.

Pratt, W. B., Morishima, Y., Peng, H. M., & Osawa, Y. (2010). Proposal for a role of the Hsp90/Hsp70-based chaperone machinery in making triage decisions when proteins undergo oxidative and toxic damage. *Experimental Biology and Medicine*, 235(3), 278–289. doi:10.1258/ebm.2009.009250.

Prentice H., Modi J. P., Wu J. Y. Mechanisms of Neuronal Protection against Excitotoxicity, Endoplasmic Reticulum Stress, and Mitochondrial Dysfunction in Stroke and Neurodegenerative Diseases. *Oxid Med Cell Longev*. 2015;2015:964518. doi:10.1155/2015/964518.

Reynolds M. R,. Berry R. W., and Binder L. I. Site-specific nitration and oxidative dityrosine bridging of the tau protein by peroxynitrite: implications for Alzheimer's disease. *Biochemistry* 44: 1690-1700, 2005.

Ribeiro F. M., Vieira L. B., Pires R. G., Olmo R. P., Ferguson SS. Metabotropic glutamate receptors and neurodegenerative diseases. *Pharmacol Res*. 2017;115:179-191. doi:10.1016/j.phrs.2016.11.013.

Rizor A., Pajarillo E., Johnson J., Aschner M., Lee E. Astrocytic Oxidative/Nitrosative Stress Contributes to Parkinson's disease Pathogenesis: The Dual Role of Reactive Astrocytes. *Antioxidants* 2019, 8:265.

Rosen D. R., Siddique T., Patterson D., Figlewicz D. A., Sapp P., Hentati A., Donaldson D., Goto J., O'Regan J. P., Deng H. X., et al. Mutations in Cu/Zn superoxide dismutase gene are associated with familial amyotrophic lateral sclerosis. *Nature*. 1993;362:59.

Ross, C. A., 2004. Huntington's disease: new paths to pathogenesis. *Cell* 118, 4–7.

Saha, R. N., and Pahan, K. (2006). Regulation of inducible nitric oxide synthase gene in glial cells. Antioxid. *Redox Signal*. 8, 929–947.

Saibil, H. (2013). Chaperone machines for protein folding, unfolding and disaggregation. *Nature Reviews Molecular Cell Biology,* 14(10), 630–642. doi:10.1038/nrm3658.

Saligrama, P. T., Fortner, K. A., Secinaro, M. A., Collins, C. C., Russell, J. Q., & Budd, R. C. (2014). IL-15 maintains T-cell survival via S-nitrosylation-mediated inhibition of caspase-3. *Cell Death & Differentiation,* 21(6), 904–914. doi:10.1038/cdd.2014.10

Sarkar, S., Korolchuk, V. I., Renna, M., Imarisio, S., Fleming, A., Williams, A., Rubinsztein, D. C. (2011). Complex Inhibitory Effects of Nitric Oxide on Autophagy. *Molecular Cell,* 43(1), 19–32. doi:10.1016/j.molcel.2011.04.029.

Sasaki, M., Gonzalez-Zulueta, M., Huang, H., Herring, W. J., Ahn, S., Ginty, D. D., Dawson, V. L., Dawson, T. M., 2000. Dynamic regulation ofneuronal NO synthase transcription by calcium influx through a CREBfamily transcription factor-dependent mechanism. *Proc. Natl. Acad. Sci. USA.* 97, 8617–8622.

Schröder M., Kaufman R. J. The mammalian unfolded protein response. *Annu Rev Biochem.* 2005; *74*: 739–789.

Singh S. Updates on Versatile Role of Putative Gasotransmitter Nitric Oxide: Culprit in Neurodegenerative Disease Pathology [published online ahead of print, 2020 Jul 23]. *ACS Chem Neurosci.* 2020;10.1021/acschemneuro.0c00230.

Singh, S. (2020). Updates on versatile role of putative gasotransmitter nitric oxide: culprit in neurodegenerative disease pathology. *ACS Chemical Neuroscience.* doi:10.1021/acschemneuro.0c00230.

Singh, S. K., Bencsik-Theilen, A., Mladenov, E., Jakob, B., Taucher-Scholz, G., & Iliakis, G. (2013). Reduced contribution of thermally labile sugar lesions to DNA double strand break formation after exposure to heavy ions. *Radiation Oncology,* 8(1), 77. doi:10.1186/1748-717x-8-77.

Singh, S., & Dikshit, M. (2007). Apoptotic neuronal death in Parkinson's disease: Involvement of nitric oxide. *Brain Research Reviews,* 54(2), 233–250. doi:10.1016/j.brainresrev.2007.02.001

Singh, S., & Dikshit, M. (2007). Apoptotic neuronal death in Parkinson's disease: Involvement of nitric oxide. *Brain Research Reviews,* 54(2), 233–250. doi:10.1016/j.brainresrev.2007.02.001

Sobrevia L., Ooi L., Ryan S., Steinert J. R. Nitric Oxide: A Regulator of Cellular Function in Health and Disease. *Oxid Med Cell Longev.* 2016; 2016:9782346. doi:10.1155/2016/9782346.

Socco, S., Bovee, R. C., Palczewski, M. B., Hickok, J. R., & Thomas, D. D. (2017). Epigenetics: The third pillar of nitric oxide signaling. *Pharmacological Research*, 121, 52–58. doi:10.1016/j.phrs.2017.04.011.

Steffan, J. S., Kazantsev, A., Spasic-Boskovic, O., Greenwald, M., Zhu, Y. Z.,Gohler, H.,Wanker, E. E., Bates, G. P., Housman, D. E., Thompson, L. M.,2000. The Huntington's disease protein interacts with p53 and CREBbindingprotein and represses transcription. *Proc. Natl. Acad. Sci. USA*. 97, 6763–6768.

Stepien, K. M., Heaton, R., Rankin, S., Murphy, A., Bentley, J., Sexton, D., & Hargreaves, I. P. (2017). Evidence of Oxidative Stress and Secondary Mitochondrial Dysfunction in Metabolic and Non-Metabolic Disorders. *Journal of Clinical Medicine*, 6(7), 71. doi:10.3390/jcm6070071.

Stewart, V. C., Sharpe, M. A., Clark, J. B., & Heales, S. J. R. (2002). Astrocyte-Derived Nitric Oxide Causes Both Reversible and Irreversible Damage to the Neuronal Mitochondrial Respiratory Chain. *Journal of Neurochemistry*, 75(2), 694–700. doi:10.1046/j.1471-4159.2000.0750694.x.

Swanson, R., Ying, W., & Kauppinen, T. (2004). Astrocyte Influences on Ischemic Neuronal Death. *Current Molecular Medicine*, 4(2), 193–205. doi:10.2174/1566524043479918.5

Tai, H. C., & Schuman, E. M. (2008). Ubiquitin, the proteasome and protein degradation in neuronal function and dysfunction. *Nature Reviews Neuroscience*, 9(11), 826–838. doi:10.1038/nrn2499.

Tegeder, I. (2018). Nitric oxide mediated redox regulation of protein homeostasis. *Cellular Signalling*. doi:10.1016/j.cellsig.2018.10.019.

Teismann, P.; Schulz, J. B. Cellular pathology of Parkinson's disease: Astrocytes, microglia and inflammation. *Cell Tissue Res*. 2004, 318, 149–161.

Tekirdag K. A., Cuervo A. M. Chaperone-mediated autophagy and endosomal microautophagy: joint by a chaperone. *J. Biol. Chem*. 2017.

Tengan, C. H., & Moraes, C. T. (2017). NO control of mitochondrial function in normal and transformed cells. *Biochimica et Biophysica Acta*

(BBA) - Bioenergetics, 1858(8), 573–581. doi:10.1016/j.bbabio.2017.02.009.

Thippeswamy, T., McKay, J. S., & Morris, R. (2001). Bax and caspases are inhibited by endogenous nitric oxide in dorsal root ganglion neuronsin vitro. *European Journal of Neuroscience*, 14(8), 1229–1236. doi:10.1046/j.0953-816x.2001.01752.x.

Tiwari, S., & Singh, S. (2020). Reciprocal Upshot of Nitric Oxide, Endoplasmic Reticulum Stress, and Ubiquitin Proteasome System in Parkinson's Disease Pathology. *The Neuroscientist*, 10738 5842094221. doi:10.1177/1073858420942211.

Tonazzi A., Giangregorio N., Console L., De Palma A., and Indiveri C. Nitric oxide inhibits the mitochondrial carnitine/acylcarnitine carrier through reversible S-nitrosylation of cysteine 136. *Biochim Biophys Acta Bioenerg* 1858: 475-482, 2017.

Uddin, M. S., Tewari, D., Sharma, G., Kabir, M. T., Barreto, G. E., Bin-Jumah, M. N., Ashraf, G. M. (2020). Molecular Mechanisms of ER Stress and UPR in the Pathogenesis of Alzheimer's Disease. *Molecular Neurobiology*. doi:10.1007/s12035-020-01929-y .

Uehara T., Nakamura T., Yao D., Shi Z. Q., Gu Z., Ma Y., Masliah E., Nomura Y., Lipton S. A. S-nitrosylated protein-disulphide isomerase links protein misfolding to neurodegeneration. *Nature*. 2006;441(7092):513–517.

Umeno, A.; Biju, V.; Yoshida, Y. *In vivo* ROS production and use of oxidative stress-derived biomarkers to detect the onset of diseases such as Alzheimer's disease, Parkinson's disease, and diabetes. *Free Radic. Res.* 2017, 51, 413–427.

Valle, C., & Carrì, M. T. (2017). Cysteine Modifications in the Pathogenesis of ALS. *Frontiers in Molecular Neuroscience*, 10. doi:10.3389/fnmol.2017.00005

Vasudevan D., Bovee R. C., Thomas D. D. Nitric oxide, the new architect of epigenetic landscapes. *Nitric Oxide*. 2016;59:54-62. doi:10.1016/j.niox.2016.08.002.

Verheij, M., Bose, R., Hua Lin, X., Yao, B., Jarvis, W. D., Grant, S., Kolesnick, R. N. (1996). Requirement for ceramide-initiated

SAPK/JNK signalling in stress-induced apoptosis. *Nature,* 380(6569), 75–79. doi:10.1038/380075a0.

Vonsattel, J. P., Myers, R. H., Stevens, T. J., Ferrante, R. J., Bird, E. D., Richardson Jr., E. P., 1985. Neuropathological classification of Huntington'sdisease. *J. Neuropathol. Exp. Neurol.* 44, 559–577.

Walker, A. K., Farg, M. A., Bye, C. R., McLean, C. A., Horne, M. K., & Atkin, J. D. (2009). Protein disulphide isomerase protects against protein aggregation and is S-nitrosylated in amyotrophic lateral sclerosis. *Brain,* 133(1), 105–116. doi:10.1093/brain/awp267.

Wang K., Liu J. Q., Zhong T., et al. Phase Separation and Cytotoxicity of Tau are Modulated by Protein Disulfide Isomerase and S-nitrosylation of this Molecular Chaperone. *J Mol Biol.* 2020;432(7):2141-2163. doi:10.1016/j.jmb.2020.02.013.

Wang, L., Hagemann, T. L., Kalwa, H., Michel, T., Messing, A., & Feany, M. B. (2015). Nitric oxide mediates glial-induced neurodegeneration in Alexander disease. *Nature Communications,* 6(1). doi:10.1038/ncomms9966.

Wang, X., Zhou, S., Ding, X., Ma, M., Zhang, J., Zhou, Y., Teng, J. (2015). Activation of ER Stress and Autophagy Induced by TDP-43 A315T as Pathogenic Mechanism and the Corresponding Histological Changes in Skin as Potential Biomarker for ALS with the Mutation. *International Journal of Biological Sciences,* 11(10), 1140–1149. doi:10.7150/ijbs.12657.

Xu Q., Hu Y., Kleindienst R., Wick G. Nitric oxide induces heat-shock protein 70 expression in vascular smooth muscle cells via activation of heat shock factor 1. *J Clin Invest.* 1997;100(5):1089-1097. doi:10.1172/JCI119619.

Yuan, H., Perry, C. N., Huang, C., Iwai-Kanai, E., Carreira, R. S., Glembotski, C. C., & Gottlieb, R. A. (2009). LPS-induced autophagy is mediated by oxidative signaling in cardiomyocytes and is associated with cytoprotection. *American Journal of Physiology-Heart and Circulatory Physiology,* 296(2), H470–H479. doi:10.1152/ajpheart.01051.2008.

Yuste, J. E., Tarragon, E., Campuzano, C. M., & Ros-Bernal, F. (2015). Implications of glial nitric oxide in neurodegenerative diseases. *Frontiers in Cellular Neuroscience,* 9. doi:10.3389/fncel.2015.00322.

Zeron, M. M., Fernandes, H. B., Krebs, C., Shehadeh, J., Wellington, C. L.,Leavitt, B. R., Baimbridge, K. G., Hayden, M. R., Raymond, L. A., 2004. Potentiation of NMDA receptor-mediated excitotoxicity linked withintrinsic apoptotic pathway in YAC transgenic mouse model of Huntington'sdisease. *Mol. Cell Neurosci.* 25, 469–479.

Zeron, M. M., Fernandes, H. B., Krebs, C., Shehadeh, J., Wellington, C. L., Leavitt, B. R., Baimbridge, K. G., Hayden, M. R., Raymond, L. A., 2004. Potentiation of NMDA receptor-mediated excitotoxicity linked within trinsic apoptotic pathway in YAC transgenic mouse model of Huntington's disease. *Mol. Cell Neurosci.* 25, 469–479.

Zhang N., Diao Y., Hua R., et al. Nitric oxide-mediated pathways and its role in the degenerative diseases. *Front Biosci* (Landmark Ed). 2017; 22:824-834. Published 2017 Jan 1. doi:10.2741/4519.

Zhang Z., Liu L., Jiang X., Zhai S., and Xing D. The Essential Role of Drp1 and Its Regulation by S-Nitrosylation of Parkin in Dopaminergic Neurodegeneration: Implications for Parkinson's Disease. *Antioxid Redox Signal* 25: 609-622, 2016.

In: Recent Developments in Neurodegeneration ISBN: 978-1-53618-859-2
Editor: Roger M. Howe © 2020 Nova Science Publishers, Inc.

Chapter 2

PARTICIPATION OF BRAIN ISCHEMIA IN THE DEVELOPMENT OF THE GENOTYPE AND PHENOTYPE OF ALZHEIMER'S DISEASE

Ryszard Pluta[*], *MD, PhD*
and Marzena Ułamek-Kozioł, MD, PhD
Laboratory of Ischemic and Neurodegenerative Brain Research,
Mossakowski Medical Research Centre, Polish Academy of Sciences,
Warsaw, Poland

ABSTRACT

Transient ischemia-reperfusion brain injury generated a massive neuronal loss in the CA1 area of the hippocampus, associated with neuroinflammation. This was accompanied by progressive atrophy of the hippocampus, cerebral cortex and white matter lesions. Furthermore, it was noted that neurodegenerative post-ischemic processes continued well beyond the acute stage. Rarefaction of white matter was significantly increased in animals within 2 years post-ischemia. Some rats that survived 2 years post-ischemia developed severe brain atrophy with dementia,

---
[*] Corresponding Author's E-mail: pluta@imdik.pan.pl.

which indicates active and slowly progressing neurodegeneration process. The profile of post-ischemic brain neurodegeneration shares a commonality with neurodegenerative processes in Alzheimer's disease. What is even more, ischemic brain damage is associated with the accumulation of folding proteins, such as amyloid and tau protein, in the intra- and extracellular space of cells. Here, post-ischemic alterations of protein which are connected with Alzheimer's disease and changes of their genes (*amyloid protein precursor* and *tau protein*) are presented. Recent advances in understanding post-ischemic neurodegeneration have revealed dysregulation of Alzheimer's disease associated genes such as: *amyloid protein precursor, α-secretase, β-secretase, presenilin 1* and *presenilin 2*, and *tau protein*. In this chapter, the latest evidence demonstrates that Alzheimer's disease-associated proteins and their genes play a key role in post-ischemic development of neurodegeneration with dementia. Ongoing interest in brain ischemia research has provided data showing that ischemia may be involved in the development of neurodegeneration of Alzheimer's disease genotype and phenotype, suggesting that brain ischemia can be considered as a useful model for understanding processes responsible for the induction of Alzheimer's disease.

Keywords: brain ischemia, neuropathology, folding proteins, amyloid protein precursor, α-secretase, β-secretase, presenilin 1, presenilin 2, tau protein, amyloid, phenotype, genotype, proteins, genes, dementia

INTRODUCTION

At this moment in time, ischemic stroke and Alzheimer's disease in humans create a huge burden to the healthcare system and caregivers due to the lack of causal treatment. Both disorders are one of the main causes of progressive disability and dementia worldwide (Feigin et al., 2009, Ballard et al., 2011), and the risk of ischemic stroke or Alzheimer's disease is 1 in 3 (Seshadri, Wolf 2007). With the rising ageing of population in the world, the number of people with dementia is forecasted to reach 82 million by 2030 and 152 million by 2050 (Ferri et al., 2005, Ballard et al., 2011). There are no effective causal therapies that could prevent or stop the progress of dementia in both post-ischemic brain and Alzheimer's disease. For that reason, there is a lot of pressure to improve the understanding of the neuropathogenesis of post-ischemic brain in connection with its recommended relationship with Alzheimer's disease (Pluta 2007b, Pluta et al., 2013a, Pluta et al., 2013b, Salminen et al., 2017, Pluta 2019) and to make causal treatment available (Ułamek-Kozioł et al., 2020a). It is noteworthy that more and more new experimental and clinical proofs indicate neuropathological and epidemiological links connecting post-ischemic brain with Alzheimer's disease-type phenotype and genotype. People studies have revealed that Alzheimer's disease is a risk factor for human stroke (Chi et al., 2013, Tolppanen et al., 2013) and *vice versa* (Gamaldo et al., 2006), indicating that the identical neuropathological processes may be involved in both diseases' final development. Experimental studies have also presented a synergistic link between post-ischemic brain and Alzheimer's disease, leading to an increased risk of cognitive decline and dementia development of Alzheimer's disease phenotype (De la Tremblaye, Plamondon 2011, Kiryk et al., 2011, Li et al., 2011, Cohan et al., 2015, Traylor et al., 2016, Salminen et al., 2017). The main causes of ischemic stroke in human clinic are atherosclerosis of both small and large vessels (Thal et al., 2003, Roher et al., 2004, Beach et al., 2007). Both vascular changes outlined above are associated with Alzheimer's disease, as well. At least 33% of patients with Alzheimer's disease have pathological alterations resulting from moderate or severe small vessel arteriosclerosis (Kalaria 2002). This leads to the idea that brain vascular disorders, like brain ischemia, may make different brain structures more susceptible to Alzheimer's disease neuropathology, additionally by impaired clearance of β-amyloid peptide from brain tissue (Farkas, Luiten 2001) and dysfunctional tau protein. Alternatively, post-ischemic brain and Alzheimer's disease may finally represent independent but convergent common neuropathological processes, and can therefore be expected to have common genomic and proteomic risk factors (Traylor et al., 2016, Pluta et al., 2019a, Pluta et al., 2019b).

DYSREGULATION OF AMYLOID ASSOCIATED GENES IN POST-ISCHEMIC BRAIN

In the CA1 area of the hippocampus, the expression of the *amyloid protein precursor* gene was below the control value 2 days post-ischemia (Table 1) (Kocki et al., 2015). Seven and thirty days following the episode of ischemia and reperfusion, the expression of the *amyloid protein precursor* gene was above the control value (Table 1) (Kocki et al., 2015). The expression of the *β-secretase* gene increased above the control value 2-7 days after ischemia in the CA1 area (Table 1) (Kocki et al., 2015). Thirty days post-ischemia, *β-secretase* gene expression was below the control value (Table 1) (Kocki et al., 2015). In the CA1 area, the expression of *presenilin 1* and *2* genes increased during 2-7 days after ischemia (Table 1) (Kocki et al., 2015). In contrast, thirty days post-ischemia, the expression of *presenilin 1* and *2* genes was below the control value (Table 1) (Kocki et al., 2015).

Table 1. Changes in the expression of the Alzheimer's disease-associated genes in the CA1 area of hippocampus at different times after experimental brain ischemia

Survival / Genes	2 days	7 days	30 days
APP	↓	↑	↑
BACE1	↑	↑	↓
PSEN1	↑	↑	↓
PSEN2	↑	↑	↓
MAPT	↑	↓	↓

Expression: ↑ increase; ↓ decrease. Genes: *APP*-amyloid protein precursor, *BACE1*-β-secrtase, *PSEN1*-presnilin 1, *PSEN2*-presenilin 2, *MAPT*-Tau protein.

The statistical significance of changes in expression of the *amyloid protein precursor* gene was between 2 and 30, 2 and 7 and between 7 and 30 days after ischemia (Kocki et al., 2015). The statistical significance of changes in *β-secretase* gene expression was between 2 and 30, 2 and 7 and between 7 and 30 days post-ischemia (Kocki et al., 2015). The statistical significance of changes in *presenilin 1* gene expression was between 2 and 30 and between 7 and 30 days after ischemia (Kocki et al., 2015). The statistical significance of changes in the expression of *presenilin 2* gene was between 2 and 30, 2 and 7 and between 7 and 30 days post-ischemia (Kocki et al., 2015).

In the CA3 region 2, 7 and 30 days post-ischemia, the expression of the *amyloid protein precursor* gene was above control values (Table 2) (Pluta et al., 2020). In this area of the hippocampus, *α-secretase* gene expression was below control within 2, 7 and 30 days post-ischemia (Table 2) (Pluta et al., 2020). The expression of the *β-secretase* gene was below the control value post-ischemia in the hippocampal CA3 region for 2-7 days (Table 2). In contrast, 30 days post-ischemia, *β-secretase* gene expression was above control (Table 2) (Pluta et al., 2020). In the CA3 region, expression of the *presenilin 1* gene increased for 2 -7 days post-ischemia (Table 2). Thirty days after cerebral ischemia, the expression of the *presenilin 1* gene was below the control value (Table 2) (Pluta et al., 2020). In this area, the expression of the *presenilin 2* gene was reduced for 2-7 days post-ischemia (Table 2). But thirty days after ischemia, the expression of the *presenilin 2* gene was above the control value (Table 2) (Pluta et al., 2020).

Table 2. Changes in the expression of the Alzheimer's disease-associated genes in the CA3 area of hippocampus at different times after experimental brain ischemia

Survival Genes	2 days	7 days	30 days
APP	↑	↑	↑
ADAM10	↓	↓	↓
BACE1	↓	↓	↑
PSEN1	↑	↑	↓
PSEN2	↓	↓	↑
MAPT	↓	↑	↑

Expression: ↑ increase; ↓ decrease. Genes: *APP*-amyloid protein precursor, *ADAM10*–α-secretase, *BACE1*-β-secrtase, *PSEN1*-presnilin 1, *PSEN2*-presenilin 2, *MAPT*-Tau protein.

The statistical significance of changes in expression of the *amyloid protein precursor* gene was between 2 and 7 and between 7 and 30 days post-ischemia (Pluta et al., 2020). No statistical significance was found during the entire period after ischemia in the *α-secretase* gene (Pluta et al., 2020). Statistically significant differences in the expression level of the *β-secretase* gene occurred between 2 and 30 days after ischemia (Pluta et al., 2020). Statistically significant differences in *presenilin 1* gene expression were between 2 to 30 and between 7 to 30 days after ischemia (Pluta et al., 2020). In *presenilin 2* gene statistically significant differences were between 2 and 30 and between 7 and 30 days after ischemia (Pluta et al., 2020).

Table 3. Changes in the expression of the Alzheimer's disease-associated genes in the medial temporal cortex at different times after experimental brain ischemia

Survival Genes	2 days	7 days	30 days
APP	↓	↑	↑
BACE1	↑	↓	↓
PSEN1	↓	↓	↑
PSEN2	↑	↑	↓

Expression: ↑ increase; ↓ decrease. Genes: *APP*-amyloid protein precursor, *BACE1*-β-secrtase, *PSEN1*-presnilin 1, *PSEN2*-presenilin 2.

In the medial temporal cortex, the expression of the *amyloid protein precursor* gene was below the control value 2 days after ischemia (Table 3) (Pluta et al., 2016a). In the above area, 7-30 days after ischemic injury, the expression of the *amyloid protein precursor* gene was above control values (Table 3) (Pluta et al., 2016a). The *β-secretase* gene expression was above the control value within 2 days after ischemia (Table 3) (Pluta et al., 2016a). Expression of the *β-secretase* gene was reduced in the medial temporal cortex 7-30 days post-ischemia (Table 3) (Pluta et al., 2016a). The expression of the *presenilin 1* gene was lowered below the control value, while the *presenilin 2* gene was above the control value 2 days post-ischemia (Table 3) (Pluta et al., 2016b). Seven days post-ischemia, the expression of the *presenilin 1* gene was reduced and the *presenilin 2* gene was increased (Table 3) (Pluta et al., 2016b). Thirty days post-ischemia, the expression of the *presenilin 1* gene was above the control value and that of *presenilin 2* gene below the control value (Table 3) (Pluta et al., 2016b).

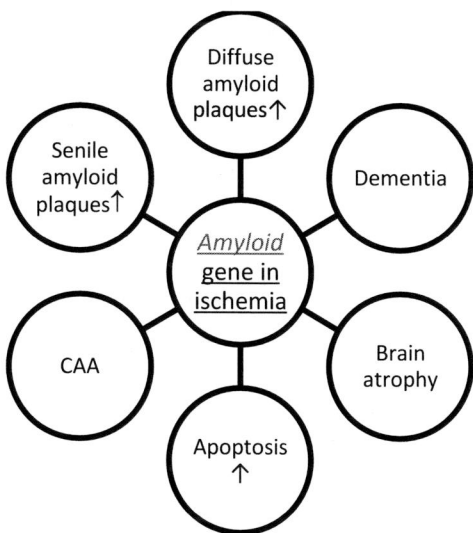

Figure 1. The role of amyloid during ischemia-reperfusion brain injury. CAA-cerebral amyloid angiopathy, ↑-increase.

For the *amyloid protein precursor* gene, its expression was downregulated 2 days after ischemia with a reverse tendency in days 7-30; significances were evident between 2 and 7 and between 2 and 30 days after ischemia (Pluta et al., 2016a). Statistically significant differences in the expression level of the *β-secretase* gene were between 2 and 7 and between 2 and 30 days post-ischemia, considering that 2 days after ischemia its expression was elevated and then moderately downregulated (Pluta et al., 2016a). There was no statistically significant difference in expression levels of the *presenilin 1* gene throughout the whole observation time post-ischemia (Pluta et al., 2016b). *Presenilin 2* gene expression was significantly elevated 2 days post-ischemia and then gradually decreased, reaching a moderate upregulation on day 7 and downregulation on day 30. Statistical significances were noted between 2 and 7 and between 2 and 30 days post-ischemia (Pluta et al., 2016b).

The results show that ischemic brain damage causes neuronal death in the hippocampus in a amyloid-dependent mechanism, defining a new and very important process that ultimately regulates neuronal survival and/or death after ischemia (Figure 1) (Kocki et al., 2015, Pluta et al., 2016a, Pluta et al., 2016b, Pluta et al., 2020).

AMYLOID IN POST-ISCHEMIC BRAIN

After experimental ischemia, with survival up to 2 years, staining to amyloid was observed in brain parenchyma. The staining was noted in intra- and extracellular space (Pluta et al., 1994b, Hall et al., 1995, Tomimoto et al., 1995, Ishimaru et al., 1996, Yokota et al., 1996, Pluta 1997, Pluta et al., 1997a, Pluta et al., 1998, Lin et al., 1999, Pluta 2000a, Pluta 2000b, Lin et al., 2001, Sinigaglia-Coimbra et al., 2002, Fujioka et al., 2003, Jabłoński et al., 2011, Pluta, Jabłoński 2012, Pluta et al., 2012a). Deposits of amyloid in extracellular space ranged from very small dots to diffuse amyloid plaques (Pluta et al., 1994b, Pluta et al., 1998, Pluta 2000a, Pluta 2000b, Pluta et al., 2000, Pluta 2002a, Pluta 2002b, Pluta 2003, Pluta 2005, Pluta 2007a, Pluta et al., 2009, Pluta et al., 2010). Diffuse amyloid plaques were documented in the hippocampus, cortex, and corpus callosum as well as around the lateral ventricles. Diffuse amyloid plaques accumulation post-ischemia in rats was not transient, since it was found out that those plaques transformed into senile amyloid plaques during long-term recirculation (Van Groen 2005). The accumulation of amyloid inside neurons and astrocytes underscores the possible importance of amyloid in the progress of post-ischemic neurodegeneration (Pluta et al., 1994b, Banati et al., 1995, Palacios et al., 1995, Yokota et al., 1996, Nihashi et al., 2001, Pluta 2002a, Pluta 2002b, Badan et al., 2003, Badan et al., 2004). In addition, these depositions may cause synaptic disintegration and turn on further retrograde neuronal death post-ischemia (Oster-Granite et al., 1996). These data indicate that post-ischemic amyloid accumulation may be responsible for extra neurodegenerative processes which could worsen the outcome during recirculation by continuous neuronal death (Pluta et al., 1997a, Pluta et al., 1997b, Pluta et al., 1998, Pluta et al., 2009, Jabłoński et al., 2011, Kiryk et al., 2011, Pluta et al., 2011, Pluta, Jabłoński 2012, Pluta et al., 2012a, Pluta et al., 2012b, Pluta et al., 2012c). Post-ischemic amyloid is generated as a product of neuronal death (Ishimaru et al., 1996). The amyloid is a neurotoxic molecule which triggers intracellular mechanisms in ischemic neuronal and neuroglial cells, which further causes additional neuronal and neuroglial cells damage or death post-ischemia (Giulian et al., 1995, Pluta et al., 2012a).

In the human post-ischemic brains the accumulation of amyloid was noted (Jendroska et al., 1995, Wiśniewski, Maślińska 1996, Jendroska et al., 1997, Qi et al., 2007). Studies demonstrated diffuse and senile amyloid plaques in the hippocampus and cortex (Jendroska et al., 1995, Wiśniewski, Maślińska 1996, Jendroska et al., 1997, Qi et al., 2007). According to another study, β-amyloid peptide 1–40 and 1–42 was documented in human post-ischemic hippocampus (Qi et al., 2007). Hippocampal and cortical neurons were the most intensely stained. Some data from a clinical study showed that blood amyloid was raised in patients post-ischemia (Lee et al., 2005, Zetterberg et al., 2011, Liu et al., 2015). The increase of amyloid in blood correlated with clinical outcome after ischemic brain episode (Zetterberg et al., 2011).

DYSREGULATION OF THE TAU PROTEIN GENE IN POST-ISCHEMIC BRAIN

A relationship has been demonstrated between hippocampal CA1 neuronal damage and *tau protein* gene expression after 10 minutes of global cerebral ischemia in rats, with survival 2, 7 and 30 days post-ischemia (Pluta et al., 2018). In CA1 neurons, *tau protein* gene expression increased above the control value on the second day after cerebral ischemia (Table 1) (Pluta et al., 2018). On the seventh and thirtieth day of recirculation after an ischemic episode, gene expression was below the control values (Table 1)

(Pluta et al., 2018). The statistical significance of changes in *tau protein* gene expression in rats was between 2 and 7 and 2 and 30 days after ischemia (Pluta et al., 2018).

In the CA3 region of the hippocampus, the expression of the *tau protein* gene after ischemia with a survival time of 2 days was below control values (Table 2) (Pluta et al., 2020). Still, 7-30 days after ischemia, *tau protein* gene expression was higher than control values (Table 2) (Pluta et al., 2020). The changes were statistically significant between days 2 and 7 and between days 2 and 30 after ischemia (Pluta et al., 2020).

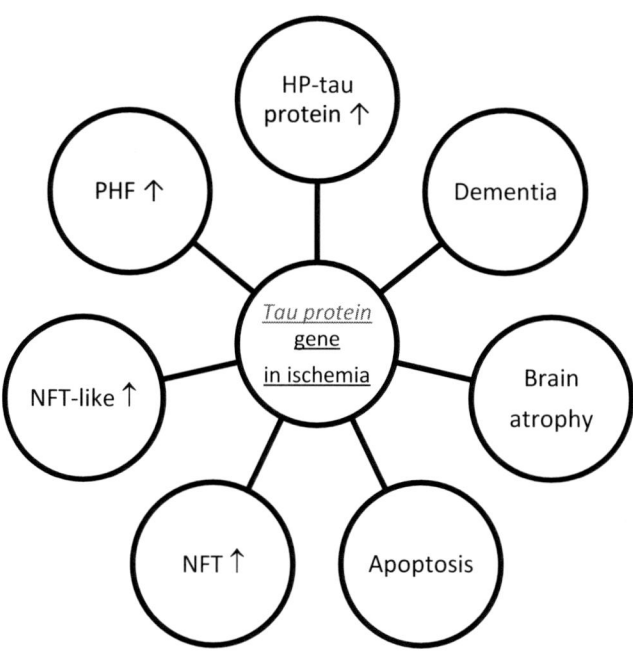

Figure 2. The role of tau protein during ischemia-reperfusion brain injury. HP-tau protein-hyperphosphorylated tau protein, PHF-paired helical filaments, NFT-like-neurofibrillary tangle-like, NFT-neurofibrillary tangle, increase↑.

The results show that ischemic brain damage causes neuronal death in the hippocampus in a tau protein-dependent mechanism, defining a new and very important process that ultimately regulates neuronal survival and/or death after ischemia (Figure 2) (Pluta et al., 2020).

TAU PROTEIN IN POST-ISCHEMIC BRAIN

Neuronal massive staining of tau protein was documented in post-ischemic hippocampus and cortex (Dewar et al., 1993, Dewar et al., 1994, Geddes et al., 1994, Sinigaglia-Coimbra et al., 2002). Furthermore, tau protein staining was found in ischemic astrocytes, microglia and oligodendrocytes (Dewar, Dawson 1995, Irving et al., 1997, Uchihara et al., 2004, Majd et al., 2016, Fujii et al., 2017). Available evidence shows that post-ischemia, hyperphosphorylated tau protein dominates in neurons and goes along with apoptosis (Wen et al., 2004a, Wen et al., 2004b, Wen et al., 2007, Majd et al., 2016, Fujii et al., 2017). The above-mentioned data point out that neuronal apoptosis post-ischemia is straightaway connected with tau protein hyperphosphorylation. Other data reveal that brain ischemia was engaged in paired helical filaments (Khan et al., 2018), neurofibrillary tangle-like (Wen et al., 2004a, Wen et al., 2004b, Wen et al., 2007) and neurofibrillary tangle (Kato et al., 1988) development post-ischemia. Tau protein was measurable in serum samples following brain ischemia and most probably indicated the progress of neuronal changes during recirculation (Bitsch et al., 2002, Kurzepa et al., 2010, Bielewicz et al., 2011, Mörtberg et al., 2011, Randall et al., 2013, Lasek-Bal et al., 2016, De Vos et al., 2017).

NEUROPATHOLOGY IN POST-ISCHEMIC BRAIN

The death of neuronal cells in the CA1 area of hippocampus develops 2-7 days post-ischemia. Extended survival after brain ischemia with reperfusion up to 2 years triggers pathology e.g., in neurons in the CA3 area of hippocampus which is resistant to ischemia (Pluta et al., 2009). On the contrary, changes in the striatum, mainly of medium-sized neurons, are found primarily in the dorsolateral region. In post-ischemic cortex, layers 3, 5 and 6 presented massive neuronal changes (Pluta 2000a, Pluta 2002a, Pluta 2002b). Between 6-24 months after brain ischemia, in addition to localized neuronal disappearance, a variety of pathological stages of neurons were noted. The first took the form of chronic neuronal change. The other changes were acute and were observed in those regions of brain, which were not involved in early pathology, e.g., areas CA2, CA3 and CA4 of the hippocampus (Pluta et al., 2009).

An ischemia-reperfusion brain episode starts a number of alterations that increase the permeability of the blood-brain barrier to non-cellular and cellular blood components (e.g., amyloid, platelets), lead to opening of tight junctions and diffuse leakage of blood components through the necrotic wall of the blood-brain barrier microvessels (Mossakowski et al., 1993, Mossakowski et al., 1994, Pluta et al., 1994a, Wisniewski et al., 1995, Pluta 2005, Pluta et al., 2006). In ischemic insufficiency of the blood-brain barrier, two unusual features deserve attention. The first is important because of the chronic effects of extravasated amyloid (Pluta et al., 1996, Pluta et al., 1997b) in the progress of neurodegeneration, and the other relates to the leakage of platelets containing huge amount of amyloid, which causes toxic, mechanical, and rapid damage of brain tissue (Pluta et al., 1994c). The ability of the amyloid to go across the ischemic blood-brain barrier leads to its influence of neurotoxic effects on specific neuronal populations, which may then lead to subsequent increased generation of amyloid in brain. Soluble amyloid is delivered to post-ischemic brain and its circulation, and as a result it contributes to the development of brain amyloidosis, vasoconstriction and cerebral amyloid angiopathy after an ischemic-reperfusion brain injury (Jendroska et al., 1995, Wiśniewski et al., 1995, Pluta et al., 1996, Wiśniewski, Maślińska 1996, Jendroska et al., 1997, Pluta et al., 1999, Lee et al., 2005, Qi et al., 2007, Zetterberg et al., 2011, Liu et al., 2015).

In the structures of the brain with massive post-ischemic neuronal pathology, an intense neuroinflammatory response was documented (Orzyłowska et al., 1999, Pluta 2000a, Pluta 2002a, Pluta 2002b, Sekeljic et al., 2012, Radenovic et al., 2020). These evidences indicate that the rise of inflammatory factors in astrocytes and microglia is directly related to the selective sensitivity of neurons to ischemic episode (Orzyłowska et al., 1999). Post-ischemic neuroinflammatory mediators can initiate a self-sustaining cycle that leads after ischemia brain to neurodegeneration. Post-ischemia interleukin-1 is a key player stimulating neurons to amyloido-genic metabolism of the amyloid protein precursor along with the release of neuroinflammatory mediators. These processes trigger abnormality in the functioning of neurons and their death, with irreversible disruption of the neural network. Additionally, this pathology activates microglia, which leads to self-propagation of the neuroinflammatory cycle. What is more, strong evidence was provided that the amyloid, which is produced post-ischemia (Pluta et al., 1994b, Pluta et al., 2009), promotes the release of neuroinflammatory factors through microglia. In the hippocampus, activation of neuroglial cells precedes neuronal injury and their death, and lasts long after an ischemic injury (Sekeljic et al., 2012, Radenovic et al., 2020).

Mediators released by astrocytes, e.g., interleukin-1β and matrix metalloproteinases increase the permeability of the blood-brain barrier and augment the transfer of leukocytes from the blood to the brain tissue (Amantea et al., 2015). The influx of these cells leads to further post-ischemic tissue damage (Sekeljic et al., 2012, Radenovic et al., 2020). Microglia, like astrocytes, also belong to the first line of defense and are activated within a few minutes post-ischemia (Dabrowska et al., 2019). Increased activation is noted 2-3 days after the onset of ischemia, persisting for years after brain ischemia (Denes et al., 2007, Sekeljic et al., 2012, Radenovic et al., 2020). Microglia secrete pro-inflammatory substances such as interleukin-1, matrix metalloproteinase-9 and tumor necrosis factor α that are involved in the blood-brain barrier damage. Intensified influx of monocytes into post-ischemic brain is observed during 24 hours following ischemia as a result of additional damage to the blood-brain barrier by astrocytic and microglia inflammatory factors. An increased number of monocytes in brain is noted up to 7 days post-ischemia (Kim et al., 2014). Sooner or later, anti-inflammatory macrophages begin to dominate ischemic brain because they are necessary for healing and regeneration processes (Gliem et al., 2016). Another type of cells involved in the immune response triggered by brain ischemia with reperfusion are neutrophils which appear in ischemic brain tissue immediately after ischemia episode (Price et al., 2004). They concentrate close to the ischemic area and release pro-inflammatory cytokines, oxygen free radicals and proteolytic enzymes that begin additional destruction of injured brain (Dabrowska et al., 2019). The number of neutrophils appearing in post-ischemic brain directly corresponds to the size of the injury (Ahmad et al., 2014). Also, T and B lymphocytes infiltrate the post-ischemic brain. Ischemic brain is also penetrated by natural killer cells (Dabrowska et al., 2019). Dendritic cells are involved in the immune response after brain ischemia with reperfusion, too (Gelderblom et al., 2018). Mast cells from brain meninges and vessels also contribute to neuroinflammatory response in post-ischemic brain. Mast cells release cytoplasmic granules containing TNF-α, heparin, histamine and proteases e.g., chymase, tryptase, matrix metalloproteinase-9 and matrix metalloproteinase-2 underlying additional injury of the blood-brain barrier, brain edema and neutrophil penetration in to injured brain tissue (Strbian et al., 2006, Lindsberg et al., 2010, Dabrowska et al., 2019).

Changes in white matter with glial cell proliferation were noted in the brains of animals and humans post-ischemia with reperfusion (Pluta 2000a, Pluta 2002a, Pluta 2002b, Fernando et al., 2006, Pluta et al., 2006, Pluta et al., 2008, Pluta et al., 2009, Scherr et al., 2012, Sekeljic et al., 2012, Thiebaut de Schotten et al., 2014, Zamboni et al., 2017, Radenovic et al., 2020). Brain ischemia in animals triggers severe damage of the corpus callosum and subcortical white matter (Wakita et al., 1994, Pluta et al., 2006, Pluta et al., 2008, Pluta et al., 2009). Ischemia of the brain increases the permeability of the blood-brain barrier, allowing inflammatory cells and amyloid to penetrate from the blood to the brain, which additionally progresses lesions in white matter (Pluta et al., 1996, Pluta et al., 1997, Pluta et al., 1999, Pluta et al., 2000, Anfuso et al., 2004, Lee et al., 2005, Zetterberg et al., 2011, Liu et al., 2015).

Evidence suggests that transient brain ischemia triggers massive neuronal death in different structures of the brain (Pluta 2000a, Pluta et al., 2009, Bivard et al., 2018). These processes develop not only in the early stages post-ischemia, but also in the late periods after ischemia (Bivard et al., 2018). Over the years following ischemia, neurodegeneration processes cause generalized brain atrophy (Hossmann et al., 1987, Pluta 2000a, Pluta et al., 2009, Jabłoński et al., 2011, Bivard et al., 2018). Autopsy of brains following experimental ischemia-reperfusion injury with survival up to 2 years showed hallmarks of brain hydrocephalus and dilatation of the subarachnoid space around the brain hemispheres (Hossmann et al., 1987, Pluta 2000a, Pluta et al., 2009, Jabłoński et al., 2011). Complete hippocampus and striatum atrophy was observed (Pluta 2000a, Pluta et al., 2009).

DEMENTIA FOLLOWING BRAIN ISCHEMIA

Changes in the behavior of animals post-ischemia with recirculation were also noted (De la Tremblaye, Plamondon 2011, Kiryk et al., 2011, Li et al., 2011, Pluta et al., 2011, Cohan et al., 2015). Locomotor hyperactivity was observed in animals post-ischemia (Kuroiwa et al., 1991, Karasawa et al., 1994) as in Alzheimer's disease patients. A lengthening in ischemia time causes longer duration of motor hyperactivity, and this is correlated with an increased number of lost neurons and progressive neuroinflammation in brain (Pluta et al., 2010, Sekeljic et al., 2012, Radenovic et al., 2020). In addition, ischemic brain injury causes the loss of reference and working memory with the progress of a spatial memory deficit (Kiryk et al., 2011). The progress of the cognitive deficit develops systematically along with post-ischemic time length (Kiryk et al., 2011). Moreover, after repeated transient brain ischemia damage in animals, durable motor hyperactivity with cognitive deficits and reduced anxiety was noted (Ishibashi et al., 2006). The behavioral changes were related to the massive brain atrophy (Hossmann et al., 1987, Pluta 2000a, Pluta 2002a, Pluta 2002b, Pluta et al., 2009, Jabłoński et al., 2011, Pluta et al., 2012b, Pluta et al., 2012c). Learning and memory deficits post-ischemia irreversibly progressed and persisted forever (Kiryk et al., 2011).

The dangerous consequence of post-ischemic neuropathology in patients is slow and progressive development of dementia (Gemmell et al., 2012, Brainin et al., 2015, Mok et al., 2016, Portegies et al., 2016, Kim, Lee 2018). The occurrence of dementia after the first ischemic stroke and recurrent stroke is calculated approximately at 10% and 33-41% respectively

(Pendlebury et al., 2009). During a 25-year follow-up, the incidence of dementia has been calculated at approximately 48% (Kokmen et al., 1996). Worldwide, dementia after post-ischemic stroke happens between 5% and 50% of survivors, depending on population demographics, diagnostic criteria and geographical location (Surawan et al., 2017). In fact, it is certain that dementia after brain ischemia with reperfusion has many risk factors in common with the development of sporadic Alzheimer's disease. It is highly likely that post-ischemic brain changes may precede Alzheimer's disease dementia and cause all the consequences associated with the development of dementia in this disease entity.

CONCLUSION

This chapter presents neurodegeneration of Alzheimer's disease phenotype and genotype in post-ischemic brain such as: neuropathology, amyloid, tau protein, and their genes, which altogether play a key role in the development of dementia. It provides protein changes and their gene expression of the *amyloid protein precursor, α-secretase, β-secretase, presenilin 1, presenilin 2* and *tau protein* in rats post-ischemia in the region of the CA1 and CA3 of hippocampus and medial temporal cortex. The data demonstrates that ischemic brain injury triggers the death of neurons in the hippocampus and temporal cortex in a manner dependent on the amyloid (Figure 1). The above alterations are associated with the deposition of the amyloid in the intra- and extracellular space, and the loss of neurons with huge brain atrophy, which finally leads to Alzheimer's disease type dementia (Figure 1). It is very likely that post-ischemic generation of amyloid plaques in the brain is caused by an increased production, intensified inflow from plasma and worsening amyloid clearance from the brain. The above data suggest a direct relationship between ischemia and increased level of amyloid in the brain such as diffuse and senile amyloid plaques (Figure 1). On the basis of the presented observations it can be concluded that brain ischemia with reperfusion influences the processing of the amyloid protein precursor at both the gene and protein level, and leads to the accumulation of the amyloid in brain tissue (Figure 1).

Additionally, data showed that ischemia of CA1 and CA3 areas have an effect on *tau protein* gene expression. It can also be noted that dysregulated tau protein also takes part in neuronal death in the areas CA1 and CA3 of hippocampus (Figure 2). The existing evidence documented the formation of neurofibrillary tangles post-ischemia (Figure 2). In the support of the above data, an elevated Cdk5 level was observed following ischemic brain injury. This may suggest linking tau protein dysfunction with the onset of neuronal death in the hippocampus post-ischemia (Figure 2). The above data indicate regulation of ischemic death of neurons in the CA1 and CA3 area of the hippocampus in a manner dependent on tau protein stage (Figure 2).

The parallelism between these two diseases, at the molecular level, is remarkable. The conclusions drawn from the study of ischemia-induced Alzheimer's disease-related neuropathology, proteins and their genes which contribute to the death of neurons, the production of the amyloid with generation plaques (Figure 1), formation of neurofibrillary tangles (Figure 2), and finally development of neurodegeneration with dementia (Figures 1, 2) are essential for the development therapy of brain ischemia and Alzheimer's disease.

ACKNOWLEDGMENTS

The authors acknowledges the financial support from the Mossakowski Medical Research Centre, Polish Academy of Sciences, Warsaw, Poland (T3-RP).

REFERENCES

Ahmad M, Dar NJ, Bhat ZS, Hussain A, Shah A, Liu H, Graham SH. Inflammation in ischemic stroke: mechanisms, consequences and possible drug targets. *CNS Neurol Disord Drug Targets* 2014;13:1378–1396.

Amantea D, Micieli G, Tassorelli C, Cuartero MI, Ballesteros I, Certo M, Moro MA, Lizasoain I, Bagetta G. Rational modulation of the innate immune system for neuroprotection in ischemic stroke. *Front Neurosci* 2015;9:147.

Anfuso CD, Assero G, Lupo G, Nicota A, Cannavo G, Strosznajder RP, Rapisarda P, Pluta R, Alberghia M. Amyloid beta(1-42) and its beta(25-35) fragment induce activation and membrane translocation of cytosolic phospholipase A(2) in bovine retina capillary pericytes. *Biochim Biophys Acta* 2004;1686:125-138.

Badan I, Platt D, Kessler C, Popa-Wagner A. Temporal dynamics of degenerative and regenerative events associated with cerebral ischemia in aged rats. *Gerontology* 2003;49:356–365.

Badan I, Dinca I, Buchhold B, Suofu Y, Walker L, Gratz M, Platt D, Kessler CH, Popa-Wagner A. Accelerated accumulation of N- and C-terminal beta APP fragments and delayed recovery of microtubule-associated protein 1B expression following stroke in aged rats. *Eur J Neurosci* 2004;19:2270–2280.

Ballard C, Gauthier S, Corbett A, Brayne C, Aarsland D, Jones E. Alzheimer's disease. *Lancet* 2011;377:1019–1031.

Banati RB, Gehrmann J, Wießner C, Hossmann KA, Kreutzberg GW. Glial expression of the β-amyloid precursor protein (APP) in global ischemia. *J Cereb Blood Flow Metab* 1995;15:647–654.

Beach TG, Wilson JR, Sue LI, Newell A, Poston M, Cisneros R, Pandya Y, Esh C, Connor DJ, Sabbagh M, Walker DG, Roher AE. Circle of Willis atherosclerosis: association with Alzheimer's disease, neuritic plaques and neurofibrillary tangles. *Acta Neuropathol* 2007;113:13–21.

Bielewicz J, Kurzepa J, Czekajska-Chehab E, Stelmasiak Z, Bartosik-Psujek H. Does serum tau protein predict the outcome of patients with ischemic stroke? *J Mol Neurosci* 2011;43:241–245.

Bitsch A, Horn C, Kemmling Y, Seipelt M, Hellenbrand U, Stiefel M, Ciesielczyk B, Cepek L, Bahn E, Ratzka P, Prange H, Otto M. Serum tau protein level as a marker of axonal damage in acute ischemic stroke. *Eur Neurol* 2002;47:45–51.

Bivard A, Lillicrap T, Maréchal B, Garcia-Esperon C, Holliday E, Krishnamurthy V, Levi CR, Parsons M. Transient ischemic attack results in delayed brain atrophy and cognitive decline. *Stroke* 2018;49:384-390.

Brainin M, Tuomilehto J, Heiss WD, Bornstein NM, Bath PM, Teuschl Y, Richard E, Guekht A, Quinn T; Post Stroke Cognition Study Group. Post-stroke cognitive decline: an update and perspectives for clinical research. *Eur J Neurol* 2015;22:229-238.

Chi NF, Chien LN, Ku HL, Hu CJ, Chiou HY. Alzheimer disease and risk of stroke: a population-based cohort study. *Neurology* 2013;80:705–711.

Cohan CH, Neumann JT, Dave KR, Alekseyenko A, Binkert M, Stransky K, Lin HW, Barnes CA, Wright CB, Perez-Pinzon MA. Effect of cardiac arrest on cognitive impairment and hippocampal plasticity in middle-aged rats. *PLoS One* 2015;10:e0124918.

Dabrowska S, Andrzejewska A, Lukomska B, Jankowski M,. Neuroinflammation as a target for treatment of stroke using mesenchymal stem cells and extracellular vesicles. *J Neuroinflamation* 2019;16:178.

De la Tremblaye PB, Plamondon H. Impaired conditioned emotional response and object recognition are concomitant to neuronal damage in the amygdale and perirhinal cortex in middle-aged ischemic rats. *Behav Brain Res* 2011;219:227–233.

Denes A, Vidyasagar R, Feng J, Narvainen J, McColl BW, Kauppinen RA, Allan SM. Proliferating resident microglia after focal cerebral ischaemia in mice. *J Cereb Blood Flow Metab* 2007;27:1941–1953.

De Vos A, Bjerke M, Brouns R, De Roeck N, Jacobs D, Van den Abbeele L, Guldolf K, Zetterberg H, Blennow K, Engelborghs S, Vanmechelen E. Neurogranin and tau in cerebrospinal fluid and plasma of patients with acute ischemic stroke. *BMC Neurol* 2017;17:170.

Dewar D, Graham DI, Teasdale GM, McCulloch J. Alz-50 and ubiquitin immunoreactivity is induced by permanent focal cerebral ischaemia in the cat. *Acta Neuropathol* 1993;86:623–629.

Dewar D, Graham DI, Teasdale GM, McCulloch J. Cerebral ischemia induces alterations in tau and ubiquitin proteins. *Dementia* 1994;5:168–173.

Dewar D, Dawson D. Tau protein is altered by focal cerebral ischaemia in the rat: an immunohistochemical and immunoblotting study. *Brain Res* 1995;684:70–78.

Farkas E, Luiten PG. Cerebral microvascular pathology in aging and Alzheimer's disease. *Prog Neurobiol* 2001;64:575–611.

Feigin VL, Lawes CM, Bennett DA, Barker-Collo SL, Parag V. Worldwide stroke incidence and early case fatality reported in 56 population-based studies: a systematic review. *Lancet Neurol* 2009;8:355–369.

Fernando MS, Simpson JE, Matthews F, Brayne C, Lewis CE, Barber R, Kalaria RN, Forster G, Esteves F, Wharton SB, Shaw PJ, O'Brien JT, Ince PG. White matter lesions in an unselected cohort of the elderly: molecular pathology suggests origin from chronic hypoperfusion injury. *Stroke* 2006;37:1391–1398.

Ferri CP, Prince M, Brayne C, Brodaty H, Fratiglioni L, Ganguli M, Hall K, Hasegawa K, Hendrie H, Huang Y, Jorm A, Mathers C, Menezes PR, Rimmer E, Scazufca M, Alzheimer's disease international. Global prevalence of dementia: a Delphi consensus study. *Lancet* 2005; 366:2112–2117.

Fujii H, Takahashi T, Mukai T, Tanaka S, Hosomi N, Maruyama H, Sakai N, Matsumoto M. Modifications of tau protein after cerebral ischemia and reperfusion in rats are similar to those occurring in Alzheimer's disease - Hyperphosphorylation and cleavage of 4- and 3-repeat tau. *J Cereb Blood Flow Metab* 2017;37:2441-2457.

Fujioka M, Taoka T, Matsuo Y, Mishima K, Ogoshi K, Kondo Y, Isuda M, Fujiwara M, Asano T, Sakaki T, Miyasaki A, Park D, Siesjo BK. Magnetic resonance imaging shows delayed ischemic striatal neurodegeneration. *Ann Neurol* 2003;54:732–747.

Gamaldo A, Moghekar A, Kilada S, Resnick SM, Zonderman AB, O'Brien R. Effect of a clinical stroke on the risk of dementia in a prospective cohort. *Neurology* 2006; 67:1363–1369.

Geddes JW, Schwab C, Craddock S, Wilson JL, Pettigrew LC. Alterations in tau immunostaining in the rat hippocampus following transient cerebral ischemia. *J Cereb Blood Flow Metab* 1994;14:554–564.

Gelderblom M, Gallizioli M, Ludewig P, Thom V, Arunachalam P, Rissiek B, Bernreuther C, Glatzel M, Korn T, Arumugam TV, Sedlacik J, Gerloff C, Tolosa E, Planas AM, Magnus T. IL-23 (interleukin-23)-producing conventional dendritic cells control the detrimental IL-17 (interleukin-17) response in stroke. *Stroke* 2018;49(1):155– 164.

Gemmell E, Bosomworth H, Allan L, Hall R, Khundakar A, Oakley AE, Deramecourt V, Polvikoski TM, O'Brien JT, Kalaria RN. Hippocampal neuronal atrophy and cognitive function in delayed poststroke and aging-related dementias. *Stroke* 2012;43:808-814.

Giulian D, Haverkamp LJ, Li J, Karshin WL, Yu J, Tom D, Li X, Kirkpatrick JB. Senile plaques stimulate microglia to release a neurotoxin found in Alzheimer brain. *Neurochem Int* 1995;27:119–137.

Gliem M, Schwaninger M, Jander S. Protective features of peripheral monocytes/ macrophages in stroke. *Biochim Biophys Acta* 2016;1862:329–338.

Hall ED, Oostveen JA, Dunn E, Carter DB. Increased amyloid protein precursor and apolipoprotein E immunoreactivity in the selectively vulnerable hippocampus following transient forebrain ischemia in gerbils. *Exp Neurol* 1995;135:17–27.

Hossmann KA, Schmidt-Kastner R, Ophoff BG: Recovery of integrative central nervous function after one hour global cerebro-circulatory arrest in normothermic cat. *J Neurol Sci* 1987;77:305-320.

Irving EA, Yatsushiro K, McCulloch J, Dewar D. Rapid alteration of tau in oligodendrocytes after focal ischemic injury in the rat: involvement of free radicals. *J Cereb Blood Flow Metab* 1997;17:612–622.

Ishibashi S, Kuroiwa T, LiYuan S, Katsumata N, Li S, Endo S, Mizusawa H. Long-term cognitive and neuropsychological symptoms after global cerebral ischemia in Mongolian gerbils. *Acta Neurochir* (Suppl) 2006;96:299–302.

Ishimaru H, Ishikawa K, Haga S, Shoji M, Ohe Y, Haga C, Sasaki A, Takashashi A, Maruyama Y. Accumulation of apolipoprotein E and β-amyloid-like protein in a trace of the hippocampal CA1 pyramidal cell layer after ischaemic delayed neuronal death. *NeuroReport* 1996;7:3063–3067.

Jabłoński M, Maciejewski R, Januszewski S, Ułamek M, Pluta R. One year follow up in ischemic brain injury and the role of Alzheimer factors. *Physiol Res* 2011;60(Suppl. 1): 113–119.

Jendroska K, Poewe W, Daniel SE, Pluess J, Iwerssen-Schmidt H, Paulsen J, Barthel S, Schelosky L, Cervos-Navarr J, DeArmond SJ. Ischemic stress induces deposition of amyloid beta immunoreactivity in human brain. *Acta Neuropathol* 1995;90:461-466.

Jendroska K, Hoffmann OM, Patt S. Amyloid β peptide and precursor protein (APP) in mild and severe brain ischemia. *Ann NY Acad Sci* 1997;826:401-405.

Kalaria RN. Small vessel disease and Alzheimer's dementia: Pathological considerations. *Crebrovasc Dis* 2002;13(Suppl. 2):48-52.

Karasawa Y, Araki H, Otomo S. Changes in locomotor activity and passive avoidance task performance induced by cerebral ischemia in mongolian gerbils. *Stroke* 1994;25:645–650.

Kato T, Hirano A, Katagiri T, Sasaki H, Yamada S. Neurofibrillary tangle formation in the nucleus basalis of Meynert ipsilateral to a massive cerebral infarct. *Ann Neurol* 1988;23:620-623.

Khan S, Yuldasheva NY, Batten TFC, Pickles AR, Kellett KAB, Saha S. Tau pathology and neurochemical changes associated with memory dysfunction in an optimized murine model of global cerebral ischaemia – A potential model for vascular dementia? *Neurochem Int* 2018;118:134-144.

Kim E, Yang J, Beltran CD, Cho S. Role of spleen-derived monocytes/macrophages in acute ischemic brain injury. *J Cereb Blood Flow Metab* 2014;34:1411–1419.

Kim JH, Lee Y. Dementia and death after stroke in older adults during a 10-year follow-up: Results from a competing risk model. *J Nutr Health Aging* 2018;22:297-301.

Kiryk A, Pluta R, Figiel I, Mikosz M, Ułamek M, Niewiadomska G, Jabłoński M, Kaczmarek L. Transient brain ischemia due to cardiac arrest causes irreversible long-lasting cognitive injury. *Behav Brain Res* 2011;219:1–7.

Kocki J, Ułamek-Kozioł M, Bogucka-Kocka A, Januszewski S, Jabłoński M, Gil-Kulik P, Brzozowska J, Petniak A, Furmaga-Jabłońska W, Bogucki J, Czuczwar SJ, Pluta R. Dysregulation of amyloid precursor protein, β-secretase, presenilin 1 and 2 genes in the rat selectively vulnerable CA1 subfield of hippocampus following transient global brain ischemia. *J Alzheimers Dis* 2015;47:1047–1056.

Kokmen E, Whisnant JP, O'Fallon WM, Chu CP, Beard CM. Dementia after ischemic stroke: a population-based study in Rochester, Minnesota (1960–1984). *Neurology* 1996;46:154–159.

Kuroiwa T, Bonnekoh P, Hossmann KA. Locomotor hyperactivity and hippocampal CA1 injury after transient forebrain ischemia in gerbils. *Neurosci Lett* 1991;122:141–144.

Kurzepa J, Bielewicz J, Grabarska A, Stelmasiak Z, Stryjecka-Zimmer M, Bartosik-Psujek H. Matrix metalloproteinase-9 contributes to the increase of tau protein in serum during acute ischemic stroke. *J Clin Neurosci* 2010;17:997–999.

Lasek-Bal A, Jedrzejowska-Szypulka H, Rozycka J, Bal W, Kowalczyk A, Holecki M, Dulawa J, Lewin-Kowalik J. The presence of tau protein in blood as a potential prognostic factor in stroke patients. *J Physiol Pharmacol* 2016;67:691–696.

Lee PH, Bang OY, Hwang EM, Lee JS, Joo US, Mook-Jung I, Huh K. Circulating beta amyloid protein is elevated in patients with acute ischemic stroke. *J Neural Transm* 2005;112:1371-1379.

Li J, Wang YJ, Zhang M, Fang CQ, Zhou HD. Cerebral ischemia aggravates cognitive impairment in a rat model of Alzheimer's disease. *Life Sci* 2011;89:86–92.

Lin B, Schmidt-Kastner R, Busto R, Ginsberg MD. Progressive parenchymal deposition of β-amyloid precursor protein in rat brain following global cerebral ischemia. *Acta Neuropathol* 1999;97:359–368.

Lin B, Ginsberg MD, Busto R. Hyperglycemic but not normoglycemic global ischemia induces marked early intraneuronal expression of β-amyloid precursor protein. *Brain Res* 2001;888:107–116.

Lindsberg PJ, Strbian D, Karjalainen-Lindsberg ML. Mast cells as early responders in the regulation of acute blood-brain barrier changes after cerebral ischemia and hemorrhage. *J Cereb Blood Flow Metab* 2010;30:689–702.

Liu YH, Cao HY, Wang YR, Jiao SS, Bu XL, Zeng F, Wang QH, Li J, Deng J, Zhou HD, Wang YJ. Serum Aβ is predictive for short-term neurological deficits after acute ischemic stroke. *Neurotox Res* 2015;27:292-299.

Majd S, Power JH, Koblar SA, Grantham HJ. Early glycogen synthase kinase-3 and protein phosphatase 2A independent tau dephosphorylation during global brain ischaemia and reperfusion following cardiac arrest and the role of the adenosine monophosphate kinase pathway. *Eur J Neurosci* 2016;44:1987-1997.

Mok VCT, Lam BYK, Wang Z, Liu W, Au L, Leung EYL, Chen S, Yang J, Chu WCW, Lau AYL, Chan AYY, Shi L, Fan F, Ma SH, Ip V, Soo YOY,Leung TWH, Kwok TCY, Ho CL, Wong LKS, Wong A. Delayed-onset dementia after stroke or transient ischemic attack. *Alzheimers Dement* 2016;12:1167-1176.

Mörtberg E, Zetterberg H, Nordmark J, Blennow K, Catry C, Decraemer H, Vanmechelen E, Rubertsson S. Plasma tau protein in comatose patients after cardiac arrest treated with therapeutic hypothermia. *Acta Anaesthesiol Scand* 2011;55:1132–1138.

Mossakowski MJ, Lossinsky AS, Pluta R, Wisniewski HM. Changes in cerebral microcirculation system following experimentally induced cardiac arrest: a SEM and TEM study. In M. Tomita (Ed.), *Microcirculatory stasis in the brain*. Amsterdam, Elsevier Science Publishers B.V. 1993;pp:99-106.

Mossakowski MJ, Lossinsky AS, Pluta R, Wisniewski HM. Abnormalities of the blood-brain barrier in global cerebral ischemia in rats due to experimental cardiac arrest. *Acta Neurochir* 1994;(Suppl.)60:274-276.

Nihashi T, Inao S, Kajita Y, Kawai T, Sugimoto T, Niwa M, Kabeya R, Hata N, Hayashi S, Yoshida J. Expression and distribution of beta amyloid precursor protein and beta amyloid peptide in reactive astrocytes after transient middle cerebral artery occlusion. *Acta Neurochir* 2001;143:287–295.

Orzyłowska O, Oderfeld-Nowak B, Zaremba M, Januszewski S, Mossakowski MJ. Prolonged and concomitant induction of astroglial immunoreactivity of interleukin-1 beta and interleukin-6 in the rat hippocampus after transient global ischemia. *Neurosci Lett* 1999;263:72–76.

Oster-Granite ML, McPhie DL, Greenan J, Neve RL. Age dependent neuronal and synaptic degeneration in mice transgenic for the C terminus of the amyloid precursor protein. *J Neurosci* 1996;16:6732–6741.

Palacios G, Mengod G, Tortosa A, Ferrer I, Palacios JM. Increased β-amyloid precursor protein expression in astrocytes in the gerbil hippocampus following ischaemia: association with proliferation of astrocytes. *Eur J Neurosci* 1995;7:501–510.

Pendlebury ST, Rothwell PM. Prevalence, incidence, and factors associated with pre-stroke and post-stroke dementia: a systematic review and meta-analysis. *Lancet Neurol* 2009:8:1006-1018.

Pluta R, Lossinsky AS, Wiśniewski HM, Mossakowski MJ. Early blood–brain barrier changes in the rat following transient complete cerebral ischemia induced by cardiac arrest. *Brain Res* 1994a;633:41–52.

Pluta R, Kida E, Lossinsky AS, Golabek AA, Mossakowski MJ, Wisniewski HM. Complete cerebral ischemia with short-term survival in rats induced by cardiac arrest. I. Extracellular accumulation of Alzheimer's β-amyloid protein precursor in the brain. *Brain Res* 1994b;649:323–328.

Pluta R, Lossinsky AS, Walski M, Wiśniewski HM, Mossakowski MJ. Platelet occlusion phenomenon after short- and long-term survival following complete cerebral ischemia in rats produced by cardiac arrest. *J Hirnforsch* 1994c;35:463-471.

Pluta R, Barcikowska M, Januszewski S, Misicka A, Lipkowski AW. Evidence of blood–brain barrier permeability/leakage for circulating human Alzheimer's β-amyloid-(1–42)-peptide. *NeuroReport* 1996;7:1261–1265.

Pluta R. Experimental model of neuropathological changes characteristic for Alzheimer's disease. *Folia Neuropathol* 1997;35:94–98.

Pluta R, Barcikowska M, Dębicki G, Ryba M, Januszewski S. Changes in amyloid precursor protein and apolipoprotein E immunoreactivity following ischemic brain injury in rat with long-term survival: influence of idebenone treatment. *Neurosci Lett* 1997a;232:95–98.

Pluta R, Misicka A, Januszewski J, Barcikowska M, Lipkowski AW. Transport of human β-amyloid peptide through the rat blood-brain barrier after global cerebral ischemia. *Acta Neurochir* 1997b;70(Suppl.):247-249.

Pluta R, Barcikowska M, Mossakowski MJ, Zelman I. Cerebral accumulation of beta-amyloid following ischemic brain injury with long-term survival. *Acta Neurochir* 1998; (Suppl.)71:206–208.

Pluta R, Barcikowska M, Misicka A, Lipkowski AW, Spisacka S, Januszewski S. Ischemic rats as a model in the study of the neurobiological role of human β-amyloid peptide. Time-dependent disappearing diffuse amyloid plaques in brain. *NeuroReport* 1999;10: 3615–3619.

Pluta R. The role of apolipoprotein E in the deposition of β-amyloid peptide during ischemia–reperfusion brain injury. A model of early Alzheimer's disease. *Ann NY Acad Sci* 2000a;903:324–334.

Pluta R. No effect of anti-oxidative therapy on cerebral amyloidosis following ischemia–reperfusion brain injury. *Folia Neuropathol* 2000b;38:188–190.

Pluta R, Misicka A, Barcikowska M, Spisacka S, Lipkowski AW, Januszewski S. Possible reverse transport of β-amyloid peptide across the blood-brain barrier. *Acta Neurochir* 2000;76(Suppl):73-77.

Pluta R. Glial expression of the β-amyloid peptide in cardiac arrest. *J Neurol Sci* 2002a;203–204:277–280.

Pluta R. Astroglial expression of the beta-amyloid in ischemia-reperfusion brain injury. *Ann NY Acad Sci* 2002b;977:102–108.

Pluta R. Blood–brain barrier dysfunction and amyloid precursor protein accumulation in microvascular compartment following ischemia–reperfusion brain injury with 1-year survival. *Acta Neurochir* 2003;86(Suppl.):117–122.

Pluta R. Pathological opening of the blood–brain barrier to horseradish peroxidase and amyloid precursor protein following ischemia–reperfusion brain injury. *Chemotherapy* 2005;51:223–226.

Pluta R, Ułamek M, Januszewski S. Micro-blood–brain barrier openings and cytotoxic fragments of amyloid precursor protein accumulation in white matter after ischemic brain injury in long-lived rats. *Acta Neurochir* 2006;96(Suppl.):267–271.

Pluta R. Role of ischemic blood–brain barrier on amyloid plaques development in Alzheimer's disease brain. *Curr Neurovasc Res* 2007a;4:121–129.

Pluta R. *Ischemia-reperfusion pathways in Alzheimer's disease.* New York: Nova Science Publishers, Inc, USA, 2007b.

Pluta R, Januszewski S, Ułamek M. Ischemic blood–brain barrier and amyloid in white matter as etiological factors in leukoaraiosis. *Acta Neurochir* 2008;102(Suppl.):353–356.

Pluta R, Ułamek M, Jabłoński M. Alzheimer's mechanisms in ischemic brain degeneration. *Anat Rec* 2009;292:1863–1881.

Pluta R, Januszewski S, Jabłoński M, Ułamek M. Factors in creepy delayed neuronal death in hippocampus following brain ischemia-reperfusion injury with long-term survival. *Acta Neurochir* 2010;106(Suppl.):37–41.

Pluta R, Jolkkonen J, Cuzzocrea S, Pedata F, Cechetto D, PopaWagner A. Cognitive impairment with vascular impairment and degeneration. *Curr Neurovasc Res* 2011;8:342–350.

Pluta R, Jabłoński M. Alzheimer's factors in ischemic brain injury. In: Agrawal A (ed) *Brain injury, pathogenesis, monitoring, recovery and management*. InTech, Open Book, Rjeka, Croatia. 2012;pp:97–138.

Pluta R, Ułamek-Kozioł M, Januszewski S, Ściślewska M, Bogucka-Kocka A, Kocki J. Alzheimer's factors in postischemic dementia. *Rom J Morphol Embryol* 2012a;53:461–466.

Pluta R, Kocki J, Maciejewski R, Ułamek-Kozioł M, Jabłoński M, Bogucka-Kocka A, Czuczwar SJ. Ischemia signaling to Alzheimer-related genes. *Folia Neuropathol* 2012b;50:322–329.

Pluta R, Jabłoński M, Czuczwar SJ. Postischemic dementia with Alzheimer phenotype: selectively vulnerable versus resistant areas of the brain and neurodegeneration versus β-amyloid peptide. *Folia Neuropathol* 2012c;50:101–109.

Pluta R, Furmaga-Jabłońska W, Maciejewski R, Ułamek-Kozioł M, Jabłoński M. Brain ischemia activates β- and γ- secretase cleavage of amyloid precursor protein: significance in sporadic Alzheimer's disease. *Mol Neurobiol* 2013a;47:425–434.

Pluta R, Jabłoński M, Ułamek-Kozioł M, Kocki J, Brzozowska J, Januszewski S, Furmaga-Jabłońska W, Bogucka-Kocka A, Maciejewski R, Czuczwar SJ. Sporadic Alzheimer's disease begins as episodes of brain ischemia and ischemically dysregulated Alzheimer's disease genes. *Mol Neurobiol* 2013b;48:500-515.

Pluta R, Kocki J, Ułamek-Kozioł M, Petniak A, Gil-Kulik P, Januszewski S, Bogucki J, Jabłoński M, Brzozowska J, Furmaga-Jabłońska W, Bogucka-Kocka A, Czuczwar SJ. Discrepancy in expression of β-secretase and amyloid-β protein precursor in Alzheimer-related genes in the rat medial temporal lobe cortex following transient global brain ischemia. *J Alzheimers Dis* 2016a;51:1023-1031.

Pluta R, Kocki J, Ułamek-Kozioł M, Bogucka-Kocka A, Gil-Kulik P, Januszewski S, Jabłoński M, Petniak A, Brzozowska J, Bogucki J, Furmaga-Jabłońska W, Czuczwar SJ. Alzheimer-associated presenilin 2 gene is dysregulated in rat medial temporal lobe cortex after complete brain ischemia due to cardiac arrest. *Pharmacol Rep* 2016b;68:155-161.

Pluta R, Bogucka-Kocka A, Ułamek-Kozioł M, Bogucki J, Czuczwar SJ. Ischemic tau protein gene induction as an additional key factor driving development of Alzheimer's phenotype changes in CA1 area of hippocampus in an ischemic model of Alzheimer's disease. *Pharmacol Rep* 2018;70:881-884.

Pluta R. *Brain ischemia: Alzheimer's disease mechanisms.* New York: Nova Science Publishers, Inc.; 2019;pp:311.

Pluta R, Ułamek-Kozioł M, Czuczwar SJ. Shared genomic and proteomic contribution to brain ischemia and Alzheimer's disease: Ischemic etiology of Alzheimer's disease. In *Brain ischemia: Alzheimer's disease mechanisms.* Ed. R.Pluta. Nova Science Publishers, Inc., New York, USA. 2019a;209-249.

Pluta R, Ułamek-Kozioł M, Januszewski S, Czuczwar SJ. Common proteomic and genomic contribution to ischemic brain damage and Alzheimer's disease. In: *Alzheimer's Disease.* Ed. Wisniewski T. Codon Publications, Brisbane, Australia. 2019b;53-68.

Pluta R, Ułamek-Kozioł M, Kocki J, Bogucki J, Januszewski S, Bogucka-Kocka A, Czuczwar SJ. Expression of the tau protein and amyloid protein precursor processing genes in the CA3 area of the hippocampus in the ischemic model of Alzheimer's disease in the rat. *Mol Neurobiol* 2020;57:1281–1290.

Portegies ML, Wolters FJ, Hofman A, Ikram MK, Koudstaal PJ, Ikram MA. Prestroke vascular pathology and the risk of recurrent stroke and poststroke dementia. *Stroke* 2016;47:2119-2122.

Price CJS, Menon DK, Peters AM, Ballinger JR, Barber RW, Balan KK, Lynch A, Xuereb JH, Fryer T, Guadagno JV, Warburton EA. Cerebral neutrophil recruitment, histology, and outcome in acute ischemic stroke: an imaging-based study. *Stroke* 2004;35:1659–1664.

Qi J, Wu H, Yang Y, Wand D, Chen Y, Gu Y, Liu T. Cerebral ischemia and Alzheimer's disease: the expression of amyloid-β and apolipoprotein E in human hippocampus. *J Alzheimers Dis* 2007;12:335–341.

Radenovic L, Nenadic M, Ułamek-Kozioł M, Januszewski S, Andjus PR, Pluta R. Heterogeneity in brain distribution of activated microglia and astrocytes in a rat ischemic model of Alzheimer's disease after 2 years of survival. *Aging* 2020;12:12251-12267.

Randall J, Mörtberg E, Provuncher GK, Fournier DR, Duffy DC, Rubertsson S, Blennow K,Zetterberg H, Wilson DH. Tau proteins in serum predict neurological outcome after hypoxic brain injury from cardiac arrest: results of a pilot study. *Resuscitation* 2013;84:351-356.

Roher AE, Esh C, Rahman A, Kokjohn TA, Beach TG. Atherosclerosis of cerebral arteries in Alzheimer disease. *Stroke* 2004;35(11 Suppl. 1):2623–2627.

Salminen A, Kauppinen A, Kaarniranta K. Hypoxia/ischemia activate processing of amyloid precursor protein: impact of vascular dysfunction in the pathogenesis of Alzheimer's disease. *J Neurochem* 2017;140:536-549.

Scherr M, Trinka E, Mc Coy M, Krenn Y, Staffen W, Kirschner M, Bergmann HJ, Mutzenbach JS. Cerebral hypoperfusion during carotid artery stenosis can lead to cognitive deficits that may be independent of white matter lesion load. *Curr Neurovasc Res* 2012;9:193–199.

Sekeljic V, Bataveljic D, Stamenkovic S, Ułamek M, Jabłoński M, Radenovic L, Pluta R, Andjus PR. Cellular markers of neuroinflammation and neurogenesis after ischemic brain injury in the long-term survival rat model. *Brain Struct Funct* 2012;217:411–420.

Seshadri S, Wolf PA. Lifetime risk of stroke and dementia: current concepts, and estimates from the Framingham Study. *Lancet Neurol* 2007;6:1106–1114.

Sinigaglia-Coimbra R, Cavalheiro EA, Coimbra CG. Postischemic hypertermia induces Alzheimer-like pathology in the rat brain. *Acta Neuropathol* 2002;103:444–452.

Strbian D, Karjalainen-Lindsberg ML, Tatlisumak T, Lindsberg PJ. Cerebral mast cells regulate early ischemic brain swelling and neutrophil accumulation. *J Cereb Blood Flow Metab* 2006;26:605–612.

Surawan J, Areemit S, Tiamkao S, Sirithanawuthichai T, Saensak S. Risk factors associated with post-stroke dementia: a systematic review and meta-analysis. *Neurol Int* 2017;9:7216.

Thal DR, Ghebremedhin E, Orantes M, Wiestler OD. Vascular pathology in Alzheimer disease: correlation of cerebral amyloid angiopathy and arteriosclerosis/lipohyalinosis with cognitive decline. *J Neuropathol Exp Neurol* 2003;62:1287–1301.

Thiebaut de Schotten M, Tomaiuolo F, Aiello M, Merola S, Silvetti M, Lecce F, Bartolomeo P, Doricchi F. Damage to white matter pathways in subacute and chronic spatial neglect: a group study and 2 single-case studies with complete virtual ''in vivo'' tractography dissection. *Cereb Cortex* 2014;24:691–706.

Tolppanen AM, Lavikainen P, Solomon A, Kivipelto M, Soininen H, Hartikainen S. Incidence of stroke in people with Alzheimer disease: a national register-based approach. *Neurology* 2013;80:353–358.

Tomimoto H, Akiguchi I, Wakita H, Nakamura S, Kimura J. Ultrastructural localization of amyloid protein precursor in the normal and postischemic gerbil brain. *Brain Res* 1995;672:187–195.

Traylor M, Adib-Samii P, Harold D; Alzheimer's Disease Neuroimaging Initiative; International Stroke Genetics Consortium (ISGC), UK Young Lacunar Stroke DNA resource, Dichgans M, Williams J, Lewis CM, Markus HS; METASTROKE; International Genomics of Alzheimer's Project (IGAP), investigators. Shared genetic contribution to ischaemic stroke and Alzheimer's disease. *Ann Neurol* 2016;79:739–747.

Uchihara T, Nakamura A, Arai T, Ikeda K, Tsuchiya K. Microglial tau undergoes phosphorylation-independent modification after ischemia. *Glia* 2004;45:180–187.

Ułamek-Kozioł M, Czuczwar SJ, Januszewski S, Pluta R. Substantiation for the use of curcumin during the development of neurodegeneration after brain ischemia. *Int J Mol Sci* 2020a;21:517.

Ułamek-Kozioł M, Czuczwar SJ, Januszewski S, Pluta R. Proteomic and genomic changes in tau protein, which are associated with Alzheimer's disease after ischemia-reperfusion brain injury. *Int J Mol Sci* 2020b;21(3).
Van Groen T, Puurunen K, Maki HM, Sivenius J, Jolkkonen J. Transformation of diffuse beta-amyloid precursor protein and beta-amyloid deposits to plaques in the thalamus after transient occlusion of the middle cerebral artery in rats. *Stroke* 2005;36:1551-1556.
Wakita H, Tomimoto H, Akiguchi I, Kimura J. Glial activation and white matter changes in the rat brain induced by chronic cerebral hypoperfusion: an immunohistochemical study. *Acta Neuropathol* 1994;87:484–492.
Wen Y, Yang S, Liu R, Simpkins JW. Transient cerebral ischemia induces site-specific hyperphosphorylation of tau protein. *Brain Res* 2004a;1022:30–38.
Wen Y, Yang S, Liu R, Brun-Zinkernagel AM, Koulen P, Simpkins JW. Transient cerebral ischemia induces aberrant neuronal cell cycle re-entry and Alzheimer's disease-like tauopathy in female rats. *J Biol Chem* 2004b;279:22684–22692.
Wen Y, Yang SH, Liu R, Perez EJ, Brun-Ziukemagel AM, Koulen P, Simpkins JW. Cdk5 is involved in NFT-like tauopathy induced by transient cerebral ischemia in female rats. *Biochim Biophys Acta* 2007;1772:473-483.
Wisniewski HM, Pluta R, Lossinsky AS, Mossakowski MJ. Ultrastructural studies of cerebral vascular spasm after cardiac arrest-related global cerebral ischemia in rats. *Acta Neuropathol* 1995;90:432-440.
Wisniewski HM, Maslinska D. Beta-protein immunoreactivity in the human brain after cardiac arrest. *Folia Neuropathol* 1996;34:65-71.
Yokota M, Saido TC, Tani E, Yamaura I, Minami N. Cytotoxic fragment of amyloid precursor protein accumulates in hippocampus after global forebrain ischemia. *J Cereb Blood Flow Metab* 1996;16:1219–1223.
Zamboni G, Griffanti L, Jenkinson M, Mazzucco S, Li L, Küker W, Pendlebury ST, Rothwell PM, Oxford Vascular Study. White matter imaging correlates of early cognitive impairment detected by the

Montreal Cognitive Assessment after transient ischemic attack and minor stroke. *Stroke* 2017;48:1539-1547.

Zetterberg H, Mörtberg E, Song L, Chang L, Provuncher GK, Patel PP, Ferrell E, Fournier DR, Kan CW, Campbell TG, Meyer R, Rivnak AJ, Pink BA, Minnehan KA, Piech T, Rissin DM, Duffy DC, Rubertsson S, Wilson DH, Blennow K. Hypoxia due to cardiac arrest induces a time-dependent increase in serum amyloid β levels in humans. *PLoS One* 2011;6(12):e28263.

Chapter 3

INFLAMMATORY RESPONSE, EXCITOTOXICITY AND OXIDATIVE STRESS FOLLOWING TRAUMATIC BRAIN INJURY

Marco Aurelio M. Freire[1,], PhD and Daniel Falcao[2,†], DO*

[1]University of the State of Rio Grande do Norte, Mossoró, Brazil
[2]Virginia Commonwealth University, Virginia, US

ABSTRACT

Traumatic brain injury (TBI) is a major public health problem affecting both industrialized and developing countries worldwide (Humphreys et al. 2013). It is estimated that globally, 69 million people are affected by TBI every year. The World Health Organization predicted TBI would become a worldwide leading cause of death and disability (Hyder et al. 2007), surpassing many other diseases and treading to be the third leading cause of death worldwide by this year, 2020 (Meaney et al. 2014). The effects of TBI result in growing health and social-economic

---

[*] Corresponding Author's Email: freire.m@gmail.com.
[†] Corresponding Author's Email: dfneuro@gmail.com.

burden impacting societies throughout the world, especially low-income groups (Hyder et al. 2007). The long-term psychosocial outcomes that follow a traumatic brain injury event generate not only an impact on the quality of life of the survivors but also directly affect the lives of caretakers, and the whole family involved (Soendergaard et al. 2019). TBI knowledge has significantly increased, therefore leading to an evolving definition, better clinical categorization, and raising public awareness. Molecular and cellular processes involved with TBI have remained the focus of studies attempting to better understand associated neurochemical and metabolic responses (Prins et al. 2013). Recently, several studies investigating acute neural disorders due to both primary and secondary tissue damage following TBI have emerged. Following the primary trauma, which causes irreversible loss of tissue in the wounded area, the main secondary pathological mechanisms involve the physiological alteration in the levels of glutamate in the affected neural parenchyma that lead to excitotoxicity, inflammatory response, oxidative stress with subsequent disturbances in normal neurophysiological functions and ultimately cell death. Furthermore, studies have demonstrated that components of the inflammatory response are associated with both glial breakdown and demyelination, which are related to the increase of the functional deficits following the acute injury. This chapter aims to review the main processes associated with secondary tissue damage following traumatic injury to the nervous system. The understanding of the mechanisms related to neural tissue loss after TBI is crucial for the development of effective therapies that may help to minimize the debilitating condition experienced by the survivors.

Keywords: traumatic brain injury, functional impairment, epidemiology, healthcare system

INTRODUCTION

Acute neuropathological disorders such as traumatic brain injuries are among the leading causes of disabilities and death globally, afflicting especially children and adults of working age (DeKosky et al. 2010; Popernack et al. 2015; Dewan et al. 2018; Iaccarino et al. 2018). According to recent projections of the Global Burden of Disease (GBD), the incidence of traumatic brain injury (TBI) will rise over time due to the increase in population density and the increasing use of motor vehicles and bicycles

(GBD, 2016). TBI results in significant morbidity, mortality, and disability in both high-income and low-income countries (Smart et al. 2017; Dewan et al. 2018; Jiang et al. 2019; Pozzato et al. 2019; Ortiz-Prado et al. 2020).

Worldwide, approximately sixty-nine million individuals are affected by some form of TBI each year (Dewan et al. 2018). In the USA, more than 1.7 million people seek medical care for traumatic head or spinal cord injury annually (Coronado et al. 2011). Also, in the USA, TBI leads to approximately 235 000 hospitalizations for non-fatal injuries and 50 000 deaths (Andelic, 2013). TBI treatment, in general, requires prolonged clinical care and often includes functional rehabilitation (Rosenbaum et al. 2018). Among survivors, there is a large number who develop permanent sequelae, including functional and/or cognitive impairment (Coronado et al. 2011; Dewan et al. 2018).

The main causes of TBI in the USA are associated with motor automobile accidents, attacks with firearms, sports and recreational activities, violence, and unintentional falls (Taylor et al. 2017), which, according to the Centers for Disease Control and Prevention (CDC), resulted in almost 170 000 deaths in 2017 alone (Heron, 2019). The average cost of treatment and rehabilitation due to traumatic brain injuries in the USA alone was estimated to be approximately 76.5 billion dollars (CDC, 2019). Therefore, TBI emerges as a growing worldwide public health concern, with a severe socioeconomic burden associated (Badhiwala et al. 2019).

Tissue damages following TBI can be categorized into two sequential events: primary injury, elicited by a mechanical lesion at the instant of the trauma, inducing an immediate degenerative process associated with a physical impairment of the nervous tissue; and secondary insult, as know as secondary degeneration, caused by chemical mediators and substances released during the primary lesion, affecting regions initially spared from the primary traumatic lesion (Freire, 2012) (Figure 1). Following the primary injury, changes in tissue homeostasis occur in a few minutes, notably with the presence of cerebral edema, breakdown of the blood-brain barrier, disturbance in brain vasoregulation, and reduction of cerebral blood flow (Kaur and Sharma, 2018), with consequent impairment of the physiological function (Figure 1). However, depending on the extent of the damage, areas underlying the primary lesion and initially not directly affected end up being impacted by the release of cellular factors and inflammation, which ultimately become harmful agents that aggravate the global tissue state. Classically, several factors have been described to be involved in this process (Tator and Fehlings, 1991), including inflammation, oxidative stress, and neurotoxicity mediated by glutamate (Figure 1). Yet, despite the growing body of studies focusing on mechanisms associated with TBI progression, a multidimensional approach to outcome assessment and classification is still necessary to develop more effective treatments for this condition (Rosenfeld et al. 2012).

In the present chapter, we aim to briefly explore the main events associated with secondary tissue damage following TBI. The characterization of the mechanisms related to neural tissue loss after the primary injury is pivotal to the development of effective therapies that may help to minimize the incapacitating condition experienced by the survivors.

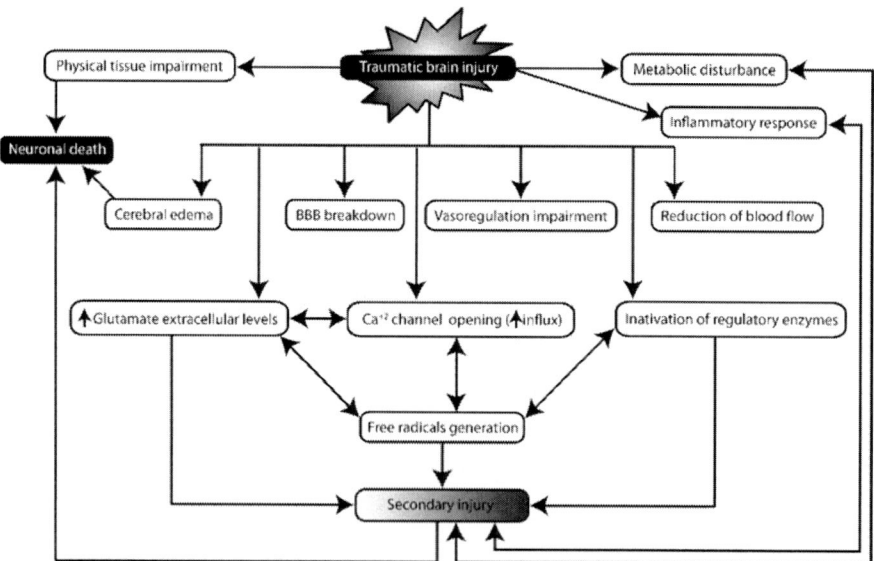

Figure 1. Summary representation of the events associated with traumatic brain injury (TBI). The primary lesion triggers a cascade of destructive events (excitotoxicity, inflammatory response, generation of free radicals, metabolism impairment) that ultimately results in cell death.

EXCITOTOXICITY FOLLOWING BRAIN INJURY

Excitotoxicity, as defined by Olney (1990), refers to the event associated with the ability of glutamate and its agonists to induce cell death when its levels are present in abnormal concentrations in the nervous tissue. In physiological conditions, extracellular glutamate concentration is strictly regulated by cellular mechanisms involving enzymes and transporters in both neurons and glial cells (Danbolt, 2001; Arundine and Timiansky, 2004). However, during TBI, these mechanisms fail in maintaining tissue homeostasis related to the concentrations of this substance in neural tissue (Choi, 1992; Karadottir et al. 2005). As a result, its concentration can rise several times above physiological conditions, becoming intolerably higher to the tissue and leading to disturbance of milieu physiology. This process elicits overstimulation of the glutamate receptors (see Figure 1), particularly NMDA receptors, and ultimately triggers both necrotic and apoptotic cell death (Choi, 1992; Gomes-Leal et al. 2004; Tehse and Taghibiglou, 2019).

A critical component in the process of cell death induced by excitotoxicity is the influx of calcium (Ca^{+2}) (Tymianski and Tator, 1996). It is known that the excessive influx of this ion into the cell is necessary for inducing neuronal degeneration. Following TBI, the binding of glutamate or its agonists to receptors of membrane specifics induces excessive excitation of neurons with an influx of Ca^{+2} many times above to physiological concentrations (Arundine and Tymianski, 2004). In addition, the mechanical force applied on the cell membranes can alter sodium influx, further activating voltage-gated Ca^{+2} channels, which can induce an influx of Ca^{+2}. The increase of Ca^{+2} intracellular levels, in turn, leads to the release of glutamate, over activating mainly NMDA receptors, which requires high levels of extracellular glutamate and membrane depolarization, conditions induced by TBI (Arundine and Tymianski, 2004) (see Figure 1).

The process of cell death by excitotoxicity involves a series of destructive biochemical cascades, which are ultimately responsible for neuronal degeneration (Choi, 1992, 1994). The neutral protease calpain, which is activated by Ca^{+2}, is known to be highly induced after activation of glutamatergic receptors (Siman et al. 1996). Calpain plays a role in degrading several structural proteins in the neuron, cleaving and inactivating the plasma membrane Na$^+$/Ca^{+2} exchanger in neurons, causing Ca^{+2} overload and necrotic and apoptotic cell death (Wang, 2000; Fricker et al. 2018).

Phospholipases, in turn, can induce rupture of the cell membrane when activated, and endonucleases can induce DNA cleavage. Ultimately, the excess of glutamate results in elevated intracellular Ca^{+2} concentrations that trigger caspase activation and production of free radicals, resulting in apoptotic cell death (Guimarães et al. 2009; Galgano et al. 2017).

INFLAMMATION FOLLOWING BRAIN INJURY

Inflammation constitutes the first line of the response of the immune system to the invasion of pathogens or in response to alterations in the tissue homeostasis. Overall, it safeguards the tissue from noxious agents and promotes healing (Freire, 2012), being commonly beneficial to the organism, by restraining the proliferation of detrimental agents, promoting restoring of the tissue, and contributing to maintaining of its homeostasis (Allan and Rothwell, 2001; Allan and Rothwell, 2003). Nevertheless, inflammation can play a dual role. In the cases of prolonged lesions or infections, chronic inflammation can release pro-inflammatory cytokines potentially cytotoxic such as interleukin 1 beta (IL-1β), tumor necrosis factor-alpha (TNF-α), transforming growth factor-beta (TGF-β), and cyclooxygenase 2 (COOX-2), which can result in impairment of both peripheral and central nervous tissue (Allan and Rothwell, 2003; Lenzlinger et al. 2001; Faden and Loane, 2015).

Evidence shows that inflammatory response may be involved in the mechanisms of secondary degeneration responsible for the exacerbation of lesions in a large number of neurodegenerative conditions, including cerebral ischemia, brain trauma, and spinal cord injury (see Figure 1). These can be characterized by substantial cell loss associated with severe functional deficits (Gomes-Leal et al. 2004; Ramlackhansingh et al. 2011).

Experimental models that induce inflammation in nervous tissue revealed the recruitment and activation processes of inflammatory cells (leukocytes and microglia) (Freire et al. 2016; Sahel et al. 2019). They also showed the increase in the expression of transcription factors that coordinate the inflammatory response in reaction to harmful conditions (Allan and Rothwell, 2001; Allan and Rothwell, 2003).

During the acute inflammatory response in the CNS, neutrophils, and macrophages are recruited to the injury site, and endothelial cells express adhesion molecules such as ICAM-1, P seletins and skeletons (Zhang et al. 1997; Schnell et al. 1999). These molecules interact with receptors found on the neutrophil membrane, which adhere to the endothelium, cross the vascular wall, and penetrate the nervous parenchyma (Dinargl et al. 1999). After neutrophil influx, monocytes migrate to the injured nerve region (Carlson et al. 1998; Dinargl et al. 1999; Raivich et al. 1999). Chemokines are synthesized by cells in the injured region and guide the migration of inflammatory cells from the bloodstream to the compromised tissue parenchyma (Carlson et al. 1998; Del Zoppo, 2000).

Microglia (macrophages resident in the CNS) plays a vital role during the inflammatory process. These cells respond quick and vigorously to the harmful insult, retracting its protractions, assuming an amoeboid shape. These cells are important phagocytes to remove cell debris and release a large number of pro-inflammatory mediators (Streit, 2000; Xiong et al. 2018).

The acute inflammatory response following TBI plays a number of benefit roles, including blood-brain barrier maintenance, debris scavenge of cytokines and neurotrophins, and immune regulation (Russo and McGavern, 2016). However, concerning long-lasting neuroinflammation, studies have stated that this condition can contribute to the impairment of the cellular environment, pointing its detrimental role in the course of tissue degeneration (Corps et al. 2015; Loane and Kumar, 2016). The reasons behind this paradoxal action still remain to be determined, but they can be related to the release of both beneficial and detrimental stimuli across specific neuroanatomical regions along the damaged milieu (Gomes-Leal, 2012; Gomes-Leal, 2019).

OXIDATIVE STRESS FOLLOWING BRAIN INJURY

Oxidative stress is one of the major contributors to the pathological condition following TBI (Abdul-Muneer et al. 2015), involving the production of derivatives of reactive oxygen species (ROS) (oxygen-free radicals and related entities such as peroxynitrite, superoxide, hydrogen peroxide, and nitric oxide) during the pathological insult, which can induce degeneration of structural and functional integrity of cells, and modification of nucleic acids, lipids, and proteins (Reynolds et al. 2007), ultimately leading to both necrotic and apoptotic cell death (see Figure 1).

Cells have a variety of antioxidant mechanisms of defense and repair against the action of these damaging substances. In some conditions, though, these systems fail, leading to oxidative stress where the production of oxidizing ROS suppresses the body's defenses because of a dysfunction in balancing the production of pro-oxidants and free radicals. In such conditions, depletion of the endogenous antioxidant system (such as decreased levels of catalase, glutathione peroxidase, and superoxide dismutase) leads to excessive ROS generation, resulting in an imbalance between oxidant and antioxidant agents that can result in neural dysfunction and death. This process is also responsible for DNA cleavage, protein oxidation, and peroxidation of cell structures, compromising the functioning of the mitochondrial electron transport chain (Chong et al. 2005).

Free radicals are extremely important for the damaging mechanisms during glutamate-mediated excitotoxic injury following TBI (Abdul-Muneer et al. 2015). ROS can induce lipid peroxidation and promote glutamate release (Agrawal et al. 2000). Activation of NMDA receptors have an important role in the formation of free radicals, in at least three ways: i) activation by Ca^{+2} of phospholipase A with the induction of the release of arachidonic acid and formation of free radicals; ii) Ca^{+2} induction of the conversion of xanthine dehydrogenase to xanthine oxidase, which is a source of free radicals (Dykens et al. 1987); iii) stimulation of NMDA receptors with a subsequent influx of Ca^{+2}, and activation of nitric oxide synthase (NOS) with NO synthesis (Dawson et al. 1991). It is believed that NO can react with the superoxide anion to produce peroxynitrite. This process can lead to the formation of potent free radicals such as the hydroxyl radical (Lipton and Stamler, 1994), and the production of NO, which performs an important role in the neurotoxicity mechanisms of glutamate. The toxic effects of NO are mainly mediated by its oxidation products, particularly the biological oxidant peroxynitrite (Pacher et al. 2007). In addition, arachidonic acid metabolism may be an essential source of free radicals as well (Choi, 1992, 1994).

There are many sources of oxidative stress after TBI, including cellular and molecular pathways that occur in several cell types, such as astrocytes and microglia, as well as injured neurons. The resultant effect of ROS production after TBI is associated with increased damage to the brain parenchyma with neuronal degeneration, increased inflammatory response, and loss of physiological functions (Lutton et al. 2019).

CONCLUSION

Traumatic brain and spinal cord injuries are the leading cause of mortality, morbidity or disability worldwide, interfering severely with the lives of the affected individuals and imposing a significant socioeconomic burden. Among the detrimental events observed in the course of a TBI, excitotoxicity, inflammation, and oxidative stress plays a pivotal role, resulting in neuronal death and consequent functional impairment, with devasting consequences. A proper understanding of the events underlying the secondary damage resulting from TBI is essential for the development of medical approaches and rehabilitation strategies appropriated that ensure a better quality of life for its sufferers.

ACKNOWLEDGMENTS

This study is part of the requirements for the Ph.D degree in Physiological Sciences (PPGMCF) of Marco Aurelio M. Freire at the

University of the State of Rio Grande do Norte - Brazil, who received a CNPq fellowship.

REFERENCES

Abdul-Muneer, P. M., N. Chandra, and J. Haorah (2015). Interactions of oxidative stress and neurovascular inflammation in the pathogenesis of traumatic brain injury. *J. Mol. Neurobiol.* 51, 966-979.

Agrawal, S. K., R. Nashmi, and M. G. Fehlings (2000). Role of L- and N-type calcium channels in the pathophysiology of traumatic spinal cord white matter injury. *Neuroscience* 99, 179-188.

Allan, S. M. and N. J. Rothwell (2001). Cytokines and acute neurodegeneration. *Nature Rev. Neurosci.* 10, 734-744.

Allan, S. M. and N. J. Rothwell (2003). Inflammation in Centrsl Nervous System injury. *Philos. Trans. R Soc. Lond. B Biol. Sci.* 1438, 1669-1677.

Andelic, N. (2013). The epidemiology of traumatic brain injury. *Lancet Neurol.* 12, 28-29.

Arundine, M. and M. Tymianski (2004). Molecular mechanisms of glutamate-dependent neurodegeneration in ischemia and traumatic brain injury. *Cell Mol. Life Sci.* 61, 657-68.

Badhiwala, J. H., J. R. Wilson and M. G. Fehlings (2019). Global burden of traumatic brain and spinal cord injury. *Lancet Neurol.* 18, 24-25.

Carlson, S. L., M. E. Parrish, J. E. Springer, K. Doty and L. Dossett (1998). Acute inflammatory response in spinal cord following impact injury. *Exp. Neurol.* 151, 77-88.

CDC - Centers for Disease Control and Prevention (2019). Surveillance Report of Traumatic Brain Injury-related Emergency Department Visits, Hospitalizations, and Deaths - United States, 2014. Centers for Disease Control and Prevention, U. S. Department of Health and Human Services.

Choi, D. W. (1992). Excitotoxic cell death. *J. Neurobiol.* 23, 1261-1276.

Choi, D. W. (1994). Glutamate receptors and the induction of excitotoxic neuronal death. *Prog. Brain Res.* 100, 47-51.

Chong, Z. Z., F. Li, and K. Maiese. (2005) Oxidative stress in the brain: novel cellular targets that govern survival during neurodegenerative disease. *Prog. Neurobiol.* 75, 207-246.

Coronado, V. G., L. Xu, S. V. Basavaraju, L. C. McGuire, M. M. Wald, M. D. Faul MD, B. R. Guzman and J. D. Hemphill (2011). Surveillance for traumatic brain injury-related deaths--United States, 1997-2007. *MMWR Surveill. Summ.* 60, 1-32.

Corps, K. N., T. L. Roth and D. B. McGavern (2015). Inflammation and neuroprotection in traumatic brain injury. *JAMA Neurol.* 72, 355-362.

Danbolt, N. C. (2001). Glutamate uptake. *Prog. Neurobiol.* 65, 1-105.

Dawson, V. L., T. M. Dawson, E. D. London, D. S. Bredt and Snyder, S. H. (1991). Nitric oxide mediates glutamate neurotoxicity in primary cortical cultures. *Proc. Natl. Acad. Sci. USA* 88, 6368-6371.

DeKosky, S. T., M. D. Ikonomovic and S. Gandy (2010). Traumatic brain injury - football, warfare, and long-term effects. *N. Engl. J. Med.* 363, 1293-1296.

Del Zoppo, G. L. (2000). Antithombotic treatments in acute ischemic stroke. *Curr. Opin. Hematol.* 7, 309-315.

Dewan, M. C., A. Rattani, S. Gupta, R. E. Baticulon, Y. C. Hung, M. Punchak, A. Agrawal, A. O. Adeleye, M. G. Shrime, A. M. Rubiano, J. V. Rosenfeld and K. B. Park (2018). Estimating the global incidence of traumatic brain injury. *J. Neurosurj.* 1, 1-18.

Faden, A. I. and D. J. Loane (2015). Chronic neurodegeneration after traumatic brain injury: Alzheimer disease, chronic traumatic encephalopathy, or persistent neuroinflammation? *Neurotherapeutics* 12, 143-150.

Freire, M. A. M. (2012). Pathophysiology of neurodegeneration following traumatic brain injury. *West Indian Med. J.* 61, 751-755.

Freire, M. A. M., J. S. Guimaraes, J. R. Santos, H. Simplicio and W. Gomes-Leal (2016). Morphometric analysis of NADPH diaphorase reactive neurons in a rat model of focal excitotoxic striatal injury. *Neuropathology* 36, 527-534.

Fricker, M., A. M. Tolkovsky, V. Borutaite, M. Coleman and G. C. Brown (2018). Neuronal cell death. *Physiol. Rev.* 98, 813-880.

Galgano, M., G. Toshkezi and X. Qiu (2017). Traumatic Brain Injury: Current treatment strategies and future endeavors. *Cell Transplant.* 26, 1118-1130.

Global Burden of Disease Study 2016. Traumatic Brain Injury and Spinal Cord Injury Collaborators. Global, regional, and national burden of traumatic brain injury and spinal cord injury, 1990-2016: a systematic analysis for the Global Burden of Disease Study 2016. *Lancet Neurol.* 2019 18, 56-87.

Gomes-Leal W. (2012). Microglial physiopathology: how to explain the dual role of microglia after acute neural disorders? *Brain Behav.* 2, 345-356.

Gomes-Leal W. (2019). Why microglia kill neurons after neural disorders? The friendly fire hypothesis. *Neural Regen. Res.* 14, 1499-1502.

Gomes-Leal, W., D. J. Corkill, M. A. M. Freire, C. W. Picanço-Diniz and V. H. Perry. (2004). Astrocytosis, microglia activation, oligodendrocyte degeneration, and pyknosis following acute spinal cord injury. *Exp. Neurol.* 190, 456-467.

Guimaraes, J. S., M. A. M. Freire, R. R. Lima, R. D. Souza-Rodrigues, A. M. Costa, C. D. dos Santos, C. W. Picanco-Diniz and W. Gomes-Leal (2009). Mechanisms of secondary degeneration in the central nervous system during acute neural disorders and white matter damage. *Rev. Neurol.* 48, 304-310.

Heron, M. (2019). Deaths: Leading causes for 2017. National Vital Statistics Reports; vol 68 no 6. Hyattsville, MD: National Center for Health Statistics. 2019.

Hyder, A. A., C. A. Wunderlich, P. Puvanachandra, G. Gururaj and O. C. Kobusingye (2007). The impact of traumatic brain injuries: A global perspective. *NeuroRehabilitation* 22, 341-353.

Humphreys, I., R. L. Wood, C. J. Phillips and S. Macey (2013). The costs of traumatic brain injury: a literature review. *Clinicoecon. Outcomes Res.* 5, 281-287.

Iaccarino, C., A. Carretta, F. Nicolosi and C. Morselli (2018). Epidemiology of severe traumatic brain injury. *J. Neurosurg. Sci.* 62, 535-541.

Jiang, J. Y., G. Y. Gao, J. F. Feng, Q. Mao, L. G. Chen, X. F. Yang, J. F. Liu, Y. H. Wang, B. H. Qiu and X. J. Huang (2019). Traumatic brain injury in China. *Lancet Neurol.* 18, 286-295.

Karadottir, R., P. Cavelier, L. H. Bergersen and D. Attwell (2005). NMDA receptors are expressed in oligodendrocytes and activated in ischaemia. *Nature* 438, 1162-1166.

Kaur, P. and S. Sharma (2018). Recent advances in pathophysiology of traumatic brain injury. *Curr. Neuropharmacol.* 16, 1224-1238.

Lenzlinger, P. M., M. C. Morganti-Kossmann, H. L. Laurer and T. K. McIntosh (2001). The duality of the inflammatory response to traumatic brain injury. *Mol. Neurobiol.* 24, 169-81.

Lipton, S. A. and J. S. Stamler (1994). Actions of redox-related congeners of nitric oxide at the NMDA receptor. *Neuropharmacology* 33, 1229-1233.

Loane, D. J. and A. Kumar (2016). Microglia in the TBI brain: the good, the bad, and the dysregulated. *Exp. Neurol.* 275(Pt 3), 316-327.

Lutton, E. M., S. K. Farney, A. M. Andrews, V. V. Shuvaev, G. Y. Chuang, V. R. Muzykantov and S. H. Ramirez (2019). Endothelial targeted strategies to combat oxidative stress: Improving outcomes in traumatic brain injury. *Front. Neurol.* 6, 10:582.

Meaney, D. F., B. Morrison and C. D. Bass (2014). The mechanics of traumatic brain injury: a review of what we know and what we need to know for reducing its societal burden. *J. Biomech. Eng.* 136(2), 021008.

Olney, J. W. (1990). Excitotoxicity: an overview. *Can. Dis. Wkly Rep.* 16 Suppl. 1E: 47-57; discussion 8.

Ortiz-Prado, E., G. Mascialino, C. Paz, A. Rodriguez-Lorenzana, L. Gómez-Barreno, K. Simbaña-Rivera, A. M. Diaz, M. Coral-Almeida and P. S. Espinosa (2020). A nationwide study of incidence and mortality due to traumatic brain injury in Ecuador (2004-2016). *Neuroepidemiology* 54, 33-44.

Pacher, P., J. S. Beckman and L. Liaudet (2007). Nitric oxide and peroxynitrite in health and disease. *Physiol. Rev.* 87, 315-424.

Popernack, M. L., N. Gray and K. Reuter-Rice (2015). Moderate-to-severe traumatic brain injury in children: Complications and rehabilitation strategies. *J. Pediatr. Health Care* 29(3), e1-e7.

Pozzato, I., R. L. Tate, U. Rosekoetter and I. D. Cameron (2019). Epidemiology of hospitalised traumatic brain injury in the State of New South Wales, Australia: A population-based study. *Aust. N. Z. J. Public Health* 43, 382-388.

Prins, M., T. Greco, D. Alexander and C. C. Giza (2013). The pathophysiology of traumatic brain injury at a glance. *Dis. Model Mech.* 6, 1307-1315.

Raivich, G., M. Bohatschek, C. U. Kloss, A. Werner, L. L. Jones and G. W. Kreutzberg (1999). Neuroglial activation repertoire in the injured brain: Graded response, molecular mechanisms and cues to physiological function. *Brain Res. Rev.* 30, 77-105.

Ramlackhansingh, A. F., D. J. Brooks and R. J. Greenwood (2011). Inflammation after trauma: microglial activation and traumatic brain injury. *Ann. Neurol.* 70, 374-383.

Reynolds, A., C. Laurie, R. L. Mosley and H. E. Gendelman (2007). Oxidative stress and the pathogenesis of neurodegenerative disorders. *Int. Rev. Neurobiol.* 82, 297-325.

Rosenbaum, A. M., W. A. Gordon, A. Joannou and B. A. Berman (2018). Functional outcomes following post-acute rehabilitation for moderate-to-severe traumatic injury. *Brain Inj.* 32, 907-914.

Rosenfeld, J. V., A. I. Maas, P. Bragge, M. C. Morganti-Kossmann, G. T. Manley and R. L. Gruen (2012). Early management of severe traumatic brain injury. *Lancet* 380, 1088-1098.

Russo, M. V. and D. B. McGavern (2016). Inflammatory neuroprotection following traumatic brain injury. *Science* 353, 783-785.

Sahel, D. K., M. Kaira, K. Raja, S. Sharma and S. Singh (2019). Mitochondrial dysfunctioning and neuroinflammation: Recent highlights on the possible mechanisms involved in Traumatic Brain Injury. *Neurosci. Lett.* 710, 134347.

Schnell, L., S. Fearn, H. Klassen, M. E. Schwab and V. H. Perry (1999). Acute inflammatory responses to mechanical lesions in the CNS:

differences between brain and spinal cord. *Eur. J. Neurosci.* 11, 3648-58.

Siman, R., D. Bozyczko-Coyne, M. J. Savage and J. M. Roberts-Lewis (1996). The calcium-activated protease Calpain I and ischemia-induced neurodegeneration. *Adv. Neurol.* 71, 167-174.

Smart L. R., H. S. Mangat, B. Issarow, P. McClelland, G. Mayaya, E. Kanumba, L. M. Gerber, X. Wu, R. N. Peck, I. Ngayomela, M. Fakhar, P. E. Stieg and R. Härtl (2017). Severe traumatic brain injury at a tertiary referral center in Tanzania: Epidemiology and adherence to Brain Trauma Foundation guidelines. *World Neurosurg.* 105, 238-248.

Soendergaard, P. L., M. M. Wolffbrandt, F. Biering-Sørensen, M. Nordin, T. Schow, J. C. Arango-Lasprilla and A. Norup (2019). A manual-based family intervention for families living with the consequences of traumatic injury to the brain or spinal cord: a study protocol of a randomized controlled trial. *Trials* 20(1), 646.

Streit, W. J. (2000) Microglial response to brain injury: A brief synopsis. *Toxicol. Pathol.* 28, 28-30.

Tator, C. H. and M. G. Fehlings (1991). Review of the secondary injury theory of acute spinal cord trauma with emphasis on vascular mechanisms. *J. Neurosurg.* 75, 15-26.

Taylor, C. A., J. M. Bell, M. J. Breiding and L. Xu (2017). Traumatic Brain Injury-Related emergency department visits, hospitalizations, and deaths - United States, 2007 and 2013. *MMWR Surveill. Summ.* 66, 1-16.

Tehse, J. and C. Taghibiglou (2019). The overlooked aspect of excitotoxicity: Glutamate-independent excitotoxicity in traumatic brain injuries. *Eur. J. Neurosci.* 49, 1157-1170.

Tymianski, M. and C. H. Tator (1996). Normal and abnormal calcium homeostasis in neurons: a basis for the pathophysiology of traumatic and ischemic central nervous system injury. *Neurosurgery* 38, 1176-1195.

Wang, K. K. (2000). Calpain and caspase: can you tell the difference? *Trends Neurosci.* 23, 20-26.

Xiong, Y., A. Mahmood and M. Chopp (2018). Current understanding of neuroinflammation after traumatic brain injury and cell-based therapeutic opportunities. *Chin. J. Traumatol.* 21, 137-151.

Zhang, Z., C. J. Krebs and L. Guth (1997). Experimental analysis of progressive necrosis after spinal cord trauma in the rat: Etiological role of the inflammatory response. *Exp. Neurol.* 143, 141-152.

BIOGRAPHICAL SKETCHES

Marco Aurelio M. Freire, PhD

Affiliation: University of the State of Rio Grande do Norte

Education:

2015-2016
Post-doctoral fellow
University of the State of Rio Grande do Norte
Mossoró, RN, Brazil

2011-2012
Post-doctoral fellow
Yale University
New Haven, CT, USA

2004-2006
PhD in Neuroscience and Cell Biology, Cum Laude
Federal University of Pará
Belém, PA, Brazil

2001-2003
Master's degree in Biological Sciences
Federal University of Pará
Belém, PA, Brazil

1996-2000
Bachelor of Science in Biology, Cum Laude
Federal University of Pará
Belém, PA, Brazil

Research and Professional Experience:
2015-Present
Assistant Professor
Faculty of Health Sciences
University of the State of Rio Grande do Norte, Brazil

2011-2012
Postdoctoral fellow
John B. Pierce Lab
Yale University, USA

2011-2012
Visiting researcher
Universidad de Chile, Chile

2006-2018
Research collaborator
Federal University of Rio de Janeiro, Brazil

2003-2004
Scientific National Development fellowship
Federal University of Pará, Brazil

1999-2000
Undergrad fellowship
Federal University of Pará, Brazil

Honors and Awards:

2019 - Certificate of Reviewing, Ecotoxicology and Environmental Safety, Elsevier

2018 - Honor Mention - XXVIII Brazilian Congress of Anatomy, Brazilian Society of Anatomy

2017 - Certificate of Outstanding Contribution in Reviewing, Neuroscience, Elsevier

2017 - Top 10% most cited PLOS ONE articles, Public Library of Science

2016 - Certificate of Reviewing, Acta Histochemica, Elsevier

2012 - Selected paper – Datasheet Blank Template, Santa Cruz Biotechnology

2010 - Honor Mention – Brazilian Society of Neuroscience and Behavior

2009 - Fellowship Award – Universidad de Chile

2008 - Honor Mention – Brazilian Society of Neuroscience and Behavior

2004 - Scholarship Award – International Institute for Neuroscienceof Natal

2000 - Academic Graduate Award – Federal University of Pará

Publications from the Last 3 Years:

1. Freire MAM, Lima RR, Nascimento PC, Gomes-Leal W, Pereira A Jr. Effects of methylmercury on the pattern of NADPH diaphorase expression and astrocytic activation in the rat. *Ecotoxicology and Environmental Safety*, v. 201, p. 110799, 2020.

2. Arrais AC, Melo LHMF, Norrara B, Almeida MAB, Freire KF, Melo AMMF, Oliveira LC, Lima FOV, Engelberth RCGJ, Cavalcante JS, Araújo DP, Guzen FP, Freire MAM, Cavalcanti JRLP. S100B protein: general characteristics and pathophysiological implications in the Central Nervous System. *International Journal of Neuroscience*, v. 19, p. 1-9, 2020.

3. Gois AM, Mendonça DMF, Freire MAM, Santos JR. *In vitro* and *in vivo* models of Amyotrophic Lateral Sclerosis: an updated overview. *Brain Research Bulletin*, v. 159, p. 32-43, 2020.

4. Fagundes NCF, Couto RSD, Brandão APT, Lima LAO, Bittencourt LO, Souza-Rodrigues RD, Freire MAM, Maia LC, Lima RR. Association

between Tooth Loss and Stroke: A systematic review. *Journal of Stroke and Cerebrovascular Diseases*, v. 29(8), p. 104873, 2020.

5. Souza MF, Medeiros KAAL, Lins LCRF, Bispo JMM, Gois AM, Freire MAM, Marchioro M, Santos JR. Intracerebroventricular injection of deltamethrin increases locomotion activity and causes spatial working memory and dopaminergic pathway impairment in rats. *Brain Research Bulletin*, v. 154, p. 1-8, 2020.

6. Costa IM, Freire MAM, Cavalcanti JRLP, Araujo DP, Norrara B, Rosa IMMM, Azevedo EP, Rego ACM, Araujo Filho I, Guzen FP. Supplementation with Curcuma longa reverses neurotoxic and behavioral damage in models of Alzheimer's disease: A systematic review. *Current Neuropharmacology*, v. 17, p. 406-421, 2019.

7. Costa IM, Lima FOV, Fernandes LCB, Norrara B, Idalina Neta F, Alves RD, Cavalcanti JRLP, Lucena EES, Cavalcante JS, Rego ACM, Araujo Filho I, Queiroz DB, Freire MAM, Guzen FP. Astragaloside IV supplementation promotes a neuroprotective effect in experimental models of neurological disorders: a systematic review. *Current Neuropharmacology*, v. 17, p. 648-665, 2019.

8. Santiago LF, Freire MAM, Picanço-Diniz CW, Franca JG, Pereira A. The organization and connections of second somatosensory cortex in the agouti. *Frontiers in Neuroanatomy*, v. 12, p. 118, 2019.

9. Freire MAM, Santana LNS, Bittencourt LO, Nascimento PC, Fernandes RM, Leao LKR, Fernandes LMP, Silva MCF, Amado LL, Gomes-Leal W, Crespo-Lopez ME, Maia CSF, Lima RR. Methylmercury intoxication and cortical ischemia: pre-clinical study of their comorbidity. *Ecotoxicology and Environmental Safety*, v. 174, p. 557-565, 2019.

10. Neta FI, Costa I M, Fernandes LCB, Cavalcanti JRLP, Freire MAM, Lucena EES, Rego ACM, Araujo Filho I, Azevedo EP, Guzen FP. Effects of Mucuna pruriens (L.) supplementation on experimental models of Parkinson's disease: A systematic review. *Pharmacognosy Reviews*, v. 12, p. 78-84, 2018.

11. Norrara B, Fiuza F, Arrais AC, Costa IM, Santos JR, Engelberth RCGJ, Cavalcante JS, Guzen FP, Cavalcanti JRLP, Freire MAM. Pattern of

tyrosine hydroxylase expression during aging of mesolimbic pathway of the rat. *Journal of Chemical Neuroanatomy*, v. 92, p. 83-91, 2018.
12. Souza MF, Freire MAM, Lucena KAA, Lins LCRF, Bispo JMM, Gois AM, Leal P, Engelberth RCGJ, Silva RH, Ribeiro AM, Marchioro M, Santos JR. Deltamethrin intranasal administration induces memory, emotional and tyrosine hydroxylase immunoreactivity alterations in rats. *Brain Research Bulletin*, v. 142, p. 297-303, 2018.
13. Pereira CM, Freire MAM, Santos JR, Guimarães JS, Florencio GD, Santos S, Pereira A, Ribeiro S. Non-visual exploration of novel objects increases the levels of plasticity factors in the rat primary visual cortex. *PeerJ*, v. 6, p. 6:e5678, 2018.

Daniel Falcao, DO

Affiliation: Virginia Commonwealth University, VA, US

Education:

2007-2011
Doctor of Osteopathic Medicine
Nova Southeastern University College of Osteopathic Medicine
Fort Lauderdale, FL, USA

2004-2006
Bachelor of Science in Biology, Magna Cum Laude, Minor in Psychology
Florida Atlantic University
Boca Raton, FL, USA

2002-2004
Associate in Arts Degree, Highest Honors and Distinction
Miami Dade College
Miami, FL, USA

Research and Professional Experience:

2016-Present
Assistant Professor
VCU School of Medicine
Virginia Commonwealth University

2016-Present
Attending Physician Virginia Commonwealth University
Department of Neurology

2016-Present
Neurosciences Medical Director of Quality Improvement
VCU Health Systems

2018-Present
Interim Medical Director Comprehensive Stroke Center
VCU Health Systems

2018-Present
Interim Vascular Neurology Division Chair
VCU Department of Neurology

2018-Present
Medical Director of the Acute Neuroscience Unit
Neurology and Neurosurgery VCUHS Hospital Floor

Honors and Awards:
2015 - Intermountain Institute for Health Care Delivery Research Scholarship, VCUHS Full Scholarship
2014 - VCU Neurology Chief Resident
2006 - FAU University Wide TALON Leadership and Achievement Award, Florida Atlantic University, Boca Raton
2005 - FAU Broward Campuses Undergraduate Owl of Year Florida Atlantic University, Boca Raton, FL

Publications from the Last 3 Years:
1. *High Reliability through Decentralized Committees,* 2019, Institute for Health Care Improvement International Symposium, Poster Presentation.
2. "Creation of a Dedicated Neurovascular Discharge Follow-Up Clinic in Assessing Its Effect on 30 Day Readmission Rates: A Quality Improvement Project." *2017 AAN poster presentation abstract Number 3660.*
3. "Seek and Ye Shall Find Fibrillations." Co-Author of Editorial for Stroke. *AHA Journal* (Stroke. 2016; 47:00-00).
4. "Optimizing prompt identification of patient's primary providers." VCU Health System Quality Improvement Project. 2015. Presented on April 28th, 2015 at the *Advanced Training Program in health Care delivery*, in Salt Lake City, Utah.

In: Recent Developments in Neurodegeneration ISBN: 978-1-53618-859-2
Editor: Roger M. Howe © 2020 Nova Science Publishers, Inc.

Chapter 4

ALL AROUND THE NOSE OF PARKINSONISM AND ESSENTIAL TREMOR

Michael G. Sadovsky[1,2,*], *Vladislav G. Abramov*[3,†],
Denis D. Pokhabov[2,3,‡], *Maria E. Tunik*[2,3,§],
Alina A. Khoroshavina[2,¶], *Ksenia O. Tutsenko*[2,‖],
Tatiana B. Anunchina[2,**], *Natalia V. Malchik*[2,††]
and *Dmitry V. Pokhabov*[2,3,‡‡]

[1]Institute of Computational Modeling of SB RAS,
Krasnoyarsk, Akademgorodok, Russia
[2]Krasnoyarsk State Medical University, Krasnoyarsk, Russia
[3]Federal Siberian Scientific Clinical Center of FMBA,
Krasnoyarsk, Russia

Abstract

We present comprehensive investigation of the combination of tremor and olfactory perception characteristics among the patients with Parkin-

---

*Corresponding Author's Email: msad@icm.krasn.ru.
†Corresponding Author's Email: excalibr@mail.ru.
‡Corresponding Author's Email: mr.lynch@mail.ru.
§Corresponding Author's Email: tsuprikova.mary.maria@yandex.ru.
¶Corresponding Author's Email: horoshavina-lina-yan@yandex.ru.
‖Corresponding Author's Email: kseniamkib@gmail.com.
**Corresponding Author's Email: kovaleva-tatiana@gmail.com.
††Corresponding Author's Email: malchiknv@mail.ru.
‡‡Corresponding Author's Email: neurodmit@mail.ru.

son's disease and essential tremor. Tremor studies bring abundant data records and the most informative have been found. Tremor data itself fail to discriminate Parkinson's disease patients from essential tremor ones; same is true for discrimination between the sick patients and control group. The combination of tremor data and olfactory dysfunction measurements was found to improve the discrimination all groups of patients. To measure the olfactory dysfunction, we used Sniffin' sticks test. It was found that the standard protocol makes the olfactory data measurements biased. To avoid the bias, we changed the protocol through the randomization of the sticks with different smells and different agent concentrations. Randomization seriously improved the data. Besides, two other subtests had been improved. The third subtest (identification) requires an implementation of unbiased and reliable reference of the smell recalling, while the standard protocol does not do it. We have carried out special investigation of the unattended knowledge of smells among patients suffering from neurodegeneration, conditionally healthy persons, and those with severe trauma. These data provides the reference set of smells (and numbers of answers, as well) to improve the third Sniffin' sticks subtest. Finally, the new hypothesis towards the inverse dependence between olfactory dysfunction and tremor is proven. This fact opens new horizons in understanding of relationship between tremor and olfactory dysfunction in developments of neurodegenerative disorders. Some further progress in olfactory measurements with respect to COVID-19 infection is discussed.

Keywords: olfactory, tremor, Parkinson's disease, essential tremor, Sniffin' sticks, clustering, differential diagnosis, prognosis, elastic map

1. Introduction

Neurological disorders make a problem for a number of people worldwide. Parkinson's disease (PD) and essential tremor (ET) are among them. Expected global PD rate is about 17 million people by 2040 (Dorsey et al., 2018). Treatment efficiency, primarily, depends on a correct differential diagnosis, which in some clinical cases makes a problem. Tremor is the common symptom both for PD and ET forcing patients to visit a doctor (Benito-Leon and Louis, 2006; Puschmann and Wszolek, 2011; Chunling and Zheng, 2016). Tremor varies in its manifestation (Puschmann and Wszolek, 2011; Chunling and Zheng, 2016). Louis and Ferreira (2010) reported that 4.6 % to 6.3 % in the population elder than 60 suffer from ET; that latter dominates among all movement disorders (Benito-Leon and Louis, 2006; Seijo-Martinez et al., 2013; Oh et al., 2014).

Rest tremor is the distinctive feature of PD. It goes down or disappears in some cases when a patient moves. On the contrary, for ET, postural-kinetic tremor is the specific feature.

However, from 10 % to 20 % of patients have no tremor as a symptom; meanwhile such akinetic-rigid form of PD is the most unfavorable due to rapid progress of cognitive impairment, in comparison to PD tremor-dominant form (Mansur et al., 2007; Benito-Leon and Louis, 2006; Puschmann and Wszolek, 2011).

Patients suffering from PD differ from ET patients in rest tremor; on the contrary, ET manifests through postural-kinetic tremor (Fedorova, 2016). Patient disabling tremor is the essential symptom for tremor-dominant form of PD. Also, it is the dominant manifestation of ET. PD patients with expressed tremor exhibit lower level of cognitive impairment (Zalyalova, 2011; Litvinenko et al., 2007).

However, AD patients do not suffer from tremor. Cognitive impairments are not peculiar for ET patients, as well (Ivanova et al., 2013). Thus, the differential diagnostics between ET and PD based on cognitive impairment evaluation is not reliable. Clinical efficiency of anticholinergics (acetylcholine blockers) prescribed by a doctor is another issue stressing the pathogenetic relation between tremor and olfactory (both for PD, and ET treatment) (Levin and Datieva, 2014; Levin et al., 2017).

This fact makes hard to diagnose correctly the disease in such situation, for a common neurologist practitioner. The clinical efficacy of anticholinergic treatment (acetylcholine blockers prescription) against the tremor both for PD patients, and ET patients is another argument to support certain pathogenetic relationships between these two diseases.

Olfactory dysfunction is stipulated to be the first manifest of PD often preceding the movement disorders. It happens due to neurodegenerative process starting in olfactory bulbs (Braak et al., 2002; Altunisik and Baykan, 2019), while it is not specific for ET. Hence olfactory dysfunction could be non-motor symptom of manifestation of PD; it is easy to detect.

Hence, it is clear that an investigation of interplay between the tremor of patients with PD and ET, and their olfactory function can help to diagnose correctly the specific type of a disease at the early stage. There are very few data on this problem. There is data only on the dependence of hyposmia, cognitive impairment and hallucinations (Chaudhuri et al., 2006; Chernykova et al., 2015).

This fact stands behind the idea to bring into power methods of differential diagnostics with examination based on determination of characteristic of odor perception, thus becoming an effective method of early differential diagnosis of both diseases; a number of studies address this issue (Fullard et al., 2017; Nielsen et al., 2018; White et al., 2016; Sui et al., 2019; Wu et al., 2016; Oppo et al., 2020; Mahlknecht et al., 2016). The data records of tremor of arms of patients along the data on their olfactory function can support the correct diagnosis at the early stage of disease. Speaking in advance, an identification of olfactory function (and dysfunction, in turn) should be clarified. Currently, there exists a series of methods to identify the olfactory (dys)function.

A study of combined effects of tremor and olfactory function brings a new hypothesis: namely,

The expression levels of olfactory function and tremor among PD patients are inversely related.

In other words, PD patients with increased tremor manifestation have better smell perception, and vice versa. This pattern of the inverse dependence between these two manifests of neurodegenerative diseases may provide improved differential diagnostics between PD and ET patients. Here we present the results verifying the hypothesis.

Besides, one needs to clarify the protocol for examination of olfactory function. Currently effective approach is claimed to be objective, while some essential questions towards the feasibility of the tests are not answered yet (see also the criticism of Sniffin' sticks test in (Eluecque et al., 2015; Mahlknecht et al., 2016)). Olfactory perception is quite subjective making a problem in evaluation of olfactory. A study of smell perception regardless a pathology, or a norm makes itself the problem, since that former has not proper lexicon (Barkat-Defradas and Motte-Florac, 2016). In spite of that, a number of attempts is made to implement smell perception data into a diagnostics and clinic practice. The feasibility of such tests is rather wide and does not focus on PD only: paper (Hugh et al., 2015) shows the feasibility of the tests for diagnostics and treatment improvement of children. Paper (Caglayan et al., 2016) shows this approach to be feasible for multiple sclerosis diagnostics. Also, these tests seem to be effective to determine the age determined neurological disorders (Masala et al., 2017).

In particular, Krismer et al. (2017) present Sniffin' sticks test implementation for diagnostics of PD; it is shown that this test satisfactory discriminates PD patients from healthy people. It should be stressed that Sniffin' sticks test is not unique in terms of the diagnostics and identification of neurological disorders; Lawton et al. (2016) provide a comparison of two core techniques used to evaluate olfactory degeneration: these are Sniffin' sticks test and the University of Pennsylvania smell identification test (UPSIT). It is rather important that these two tests are not identical from the point of view of diagnostics capability. This divergence improves the diagnostics possibilities of the approach.

Following are the aims of the chapter:

– To study the interplay between olfactory function and tremor, in patients with PD and ET.

– Using combined records on tremor and olfactory function, implement a reliable differential diagnostics protocol of these two pathologies.

– To verify the hypothesis on the inverse relation between tremor manifestation and olfactory function decay.

– To propose and discuss few innovative changes in standard Sniffin' sticks test protocol.

The key issue of this chapter is the hypothesis on the interplay between tremor and olfactory dysfunction. These two issues exhibit a kind of inverse dependence: than lower is tremor, then worse is smell perception, and vice versa. The results provided below approve this hypothesis; however, further studies are necessary to figure out the details of the dependence pattern between these two manifestation of neurological diseases.

Here we present some preliminary results on the implementation of olfactory dysfunction testing for the purposes of differential diagnostics of Parkinson's disease vs. essential tremor using the combination of olfactory testing and tremor data records. General invalidity of the first subtest of Sniffin' sticks test has been found and approved. On the contrary, the second subtest and the third subtest showed good performance in differentiation of healthy (control) population from sick one (PD patients). The second subtest effectively identifies healthy subpopulation, while gathers some healthy persons and sick ones into a cluster. Reciprocally, the third subtest yields good performance in identification of sick patients clustering them into three distinct clusters (of lower abundance), while the healthy population comprises a sparse extended cluster "deteriorated" with few sick patients. The feasibility of these tests for early diagnostics of essential tremor (ET) and discrimination of that latter from PD are discussed.

In brief, key outcomes of the paper are following:

– combination of olfactory measure with tremor records improves significantly the discrimination of PD patients from those with ET, and from healthy people;

– tremor manifestation is inverse to olfactory decay.

2. Materials and Methods

2.1. Testee Set

The testee set consists of three groups comprising the patients suffering from PD, ET and conditionally healthy people (control group). Totally, 64 people (33 men and 31 women conditionally healthy persons aged from 20 to 79 have been tested. Ten persons reported their sense of smell to be decreased, five persons claimed the sense to be increased and all other said it is normal. Seventeen persons in the set smoke (13 men and 4 women). Totally, 45 patients aged from 35 to 78 with PD have been enrolled into the study: 15 men and 30 women. Twenty three patients claimed their sense of smell to be decreased, all others said it to be normal. Two men and five women smoke. Totally, 40 patients aged from 22 to 82 with ET have been tested: 12 men and 28 women. Seven of them claimed that their sense of smell to be decreased, three persons claimed the sense to be increased and all other said it to be normal. Two men and five women smoke.

No healthy person with
– inflammatory diseases of the nasal mucosa and sinuses;
– recorded neurological symptoms and neurological diseases in medical records

have been enrolled into the control group. Any PD and ET patients having some other neurological diseases have been excluded from the study, as well.

2.2. Olfactory Testing

An examination procedure was based on extended olfactory Sniffin' sticks test ("Burghart Messtechnik"^{TM}, Germany) to determine three parameters: threshold, identification and discrimination.

The Sniffin' sticks test consists of three subtests (Nielsen et al., 2018; Morley et al., 2018; Miwa et al., 2019; Koçak et al., 2020).

Olfactory threshold determination. 16 enumerated sticks contain n-butanolin decreasing concentrations. A triplet (set of three sticks used in a probe) contains one stick with the compound, and two others free from that former. The subtest starts from exposure of the stick triplet No. 1 (with the maximal concentration of the compound) to a testee, just to get acquainted a testee to the specific smell and check whether (s)he perceives the smell, at all. Then a patient is exposed consequently with the stick triplets No 16, No 14, No 12, etc. to determine the detectable concentration of the smell.

To verify it, a testee tries the same triplet in another order of the sticks exposed, to approve the detection. A probe is stipulated to be positive, if in two sequential attempts the smell is positively detected. Next, the testee is exposed to the stick triplet with the next number (e. g., if triplet No 10 is detected, then (s)he tries the triplet No 11). If olfactory function and neurodegenerative disorders 3the testee claims to detect the smell and it is approved by control probe, the examination stops and this triplet number is recorded. Otherwise, the previous triplet number is recorded as successful recognition.

Discrimination test An ability of a patient to detect two identical smells from three proposed. Testing consists in a triplet probe, where each stick is exposed once. The test consists of 16 enumerated triplets trial. The sum of correct answers makes the score of the test.

Identification test An ability to refer a smell to four names. A patient is provided with a stick to smell it, then he sees a poster with four smell names; a patient must choose one name from those four ones. The sum of correct answers makes the score of the test.

2.3. Tremor Testing

To begin with, one must determine the specific type of tremor and choose the relevant method to detect it (Puschmann and Wszolek, 2011; Milanov, 2007; Bain, 1993). There is a number of techniques and approaches to do it. We used wireless *Colibri* instrument to monitor electrophysiological signals; four locations of sensors have been used: on the arms and forearms of both hands. Each sensor recorded three main characteristics: skin electromyogram (SEMG), gyroscope and accelerations.

To record SEMG, we placed the sensors over the tremorous muscle; upon the record of the total SEMG activity, the signal is amplified, filtered and demodulated with due procedure. The final signal represents the muscle forces both in statics, and in dynamics, as well as the fluctuations of that latter caused by tremor. Gyroscope is the sensor of angular velocities yielding the pattern of angular behavior. Also the instrument records accelerations directed along the axes of the sensors. Both amplitude and frequency of each of three characteristics were recorded. Wireless implementation allowed to register both the rest and activity values.

Tremor examination included 5 tests. The first test shows the rest characteristics. At the second test the characteristics were measure from the patients in Romberg's position. The third and fourth tests measured the characteristics when a staying patient with closed eyes was instructed to touch his/her nose tip by the left, or the right hand, respectively. Finally, the fifth test measured the tremor characteristics of a patient when he/she moved in a room. Totally 90 persons were examined, among them 30 conditionally health persons, 30 PD patients and 30 ET patients.

2.4. Statistical Methods

We used both conventional statistics methods (descriptive statistics, correlation analysis, etc.), and elastic map technique to cluster, analyze and visualize the data. The former are well described (Fukunaga, 1990; Steinley, 2010). Elastic map technique is rather novel so we describe it here in more details. Elastic map technique is a non-linear advanced statistical method to cluster, analyse and visualize multidimensional data. Mathematically, it means an approximation of multidimensional data with manifolds of low dimension.

To begin with, a dimension of the data is the number of variables (sometimes they are called *parameters* in biological and/or medical applications, while this is rather clumsy terminology). For instance, the dimension of the tremor records is 280 and the dimension of the records on Sniffin' sticks test is 52. Low dimensionality of a manifold is rather complex mathematical (topological, to be exact) concept, while we shall use manifolds of the dimension 2; further details on the topological issues of that point could be found in (Sakai, 2013; Haldane and Kosterlitz, 2016; Wang, 2012; Ault, 2018).

Manifold is another high point mathematical notion, maybe not so much familiar to medical reader. First of all, we restrict ourselves within a square and a sphere when consider various manifolds. Saying *square*, we imply a typical well-known to everyone part of a (Euclidean) plane, and a sphere might be considered as a surface of a ball. More exact (while yet not so much rigorous) a manifold is defined as an object that looks locally (in each its point) as a regular Euclidean space, while it differs from that latter globally, A square mentioned above is a trivial example of a manifold, and in such capacity it does not differ from Euclidean space.

A difference between a sphere and Euclidean space becomes clear, if one considers the behaviour of vectors established from each point of the sphere. Suppose, you take a sphere and erect a vector from each point of that latter; the vectors may be directed arbitrary. Suppose, then, you do all the same with a square. Then you take a (special mathematical) brush and "comb" all the vectors forcing them to align some definite direction. No problem takes place here, if you deal with a square.

On the contrary, a problem arises, if you try to "comb" a sphere. Indeed, all the vectors could be aligned in the specific direction, with two exclusions: these are "North polar" and "South polar". Each time you try to comb the vectors on a sphere, you find two of them that **must** be aligned into an infinite number of various directions, simultaneously. Of course, it is not possible; this impossibility makes the difference of a sphere from a Euclidean space.

Anyway, we shall constrain ourselves with square and regular two-dimensional sphere, only. Core idea of the elastic map technique is to adjust originally straight manifold to the data points, so that it fits the point "best of all". Here two questions arise:

1) What does it mean *best of all*? and
2) What does it mean *to adjust*?

We shall start to answer from the second question. *To adjust* here means to deform the manifold so that it fits the data point best of all. Almost any deformation is allowed: expansion, squeezing, bending, torsion, etc. There are two options under the prohibition in use: a glue, and a discontinuity. This constraint means the topology conservation.

Best of all means an interplay and a compromise between the proximity of the jammed manifold to the data points, and its smoothness. More rigorous definitions and concepts could be found in (Gorban and Zinovyev, 2015, 2010, 2007).

An implementation of an elastic map consists of the following six steps:

Linear preset for manifold. The procedure starts from the determination of the first and the second principal components, of the dataset. Geometrically, it consists in the search of the directions of the greatest extension of the dataset. Of course, these two directions must be orthogonal. As soon, as these principal components are found, stretch a plane over them (as on two axes).

Data projection and spring erection At the next step, each data point must be projected on the plane and the minimal square comprising all the projections must be determined. In case of a sphere, this substep should be skipped. As soon, as all the projections are determined, each data point must be connected to its projection with a mathematical spring. Such spring yields an infinite expansibility and the elasticity coefficient remains permanent, for any expansion.

Elastic membrane implementation. Next, originally rigid square (or sphere) should be substituted with an elastic membrane. The membrane is stipulated to be homogeneous: it may bend, expand or squeeze regardless a direction and/or location, and the elastic properties are stipulated to be the same, for each point of the membrane.

Adjustment of the membrane. The system constructed from the elastic membrane and the springs located to the immobile data points must be released so to reach the minimum of the total deformation energy. The deformation energy is the sum of the stretching energy of the springs, and the bending energy and the energy of other membrane deformations. Ideally, the final configuration of the jammed membrane is unique, and is completely determined by the deformation parameters (expansibility coefficients, etc.) of the springs and the membrane.

Rearrangement of the data images. As soon, as the jammed membrane reaches its final configuration, the data images on that latter must be redefined. To do it, one must find the orthogonal projection for each data point on the jammed surface. This projection is the nearest point on the jammed surface, for the point.

Inner coordinates. This is the final step to visualization. Mathematically, this step consists in the inverse non-linear transformation of the jammed membrane back into a plane, or a regular sphere. To do it, one must cut-off all the springs connecting the membrane to the dataset, and release the jammed surface coming back to a plane. Of course, the images of the data points would take new positions at this straightened manifold; this relocation is the key tool to figure out cluster structuredness, in the dataset.

2.4.1. Cluster Identification

There is a number of ways to identify clusters, either in the original dataset, or in the images dataset observed over the manifold presented in the inner coordinates. Here we have no chance even to list all the methods of clustering, some essential texts and approaches could be found in (Fukunaga, 1990; Gorban and Zinovyev, 2015, 2010, 2007; Xu and Wunsch, 2005; Fahad et al., 2014; Mittal et al., 2019); surely, it is not a comprehensive list of papers on that subject, moreover, it is rather subjective, and Reader is expected to find his/her own list of the publications of interest.

In our studies, the clusters were identified through the local density of points (see, e. g., (Halim and Khattak, 2019). To determine clusters, we supplied each image of the data point on the elastic map (presented in inner coordinates) with a bell-shaped function, e.g., Gaussian one,

$$f(r) = \mathcal{A} \cdot \exp\left\{-\frac{(r-r_j)^2}{\sigma^2}\right\}. \qquad (1)$$

It should be stressed that this choice of the bell-shaped function has nothing to do with normal probability distribution, so one should keep away from a confusion.

To determine the local density, sum up the functions (1):

$$F(r) = \mathcal{A} \cdot \sum_{j=1}^{N} \exp\left\{-\frac{(r-r_j)^2}{\sigma^2}\right\}; \qquad (2)$$

here r_j is the coordinate vector of j-th point. Then function $F(r)$ shows clusters in elastic map. Here σ is an adjusting parameter. We used freely distributed software *VidaExpert* to analyze the data. Standard soft 16×16 elastic map has been implemented, with correlation radius (see eq. (2)) $\sigma = 0.2$.

Table 1. Olfactory function investigation. stands for healthy, stands for essential tremor patients and stands for Parkinson's disease patients. Σ is the sum over three tests, n is testee number

test 1	test 2	test 3	Σ, n and percentage		
Average score ± standard deviation			Anosmia	Hyposmia	Norm
5.11 ± 2.32	11.53 ± 2.28	11.28 ± 2.18	3	32	29
			4.7 %	50 %	45.3 %
3.85 ± 2.34	10 ± 2.65	10.08 ± 2.47	2	31	7
			5 %	77.5 %	17.5 %
2.44 ± 1.91	8.76 ± 2.47	6.87 ± 2.69	14	30	1
			31.1 %	66.7 %	2.2 %

3. RESULTS

3.1. Evaluation of Olfactory Function with Sniffin' Sticks Test

We examined the olfactory functions of 45 patients suffering from PD, 40 patients suffering from ET, and 64 conditionally healthy persons (control group). That latter enrolled 33 men and 31 women aged from 20 to 79. The exclusion conditions for control group members are described above (see subsec. 2.1). In the control group, 10 persons reported their olfactory to be decreased, and 5 persons believe they have increased olfactory function. All other ones refer their olfactory as normal. 17 persons in control group (13 men and 4 women) smoke.

Patients with PD aged from 35 to 79, there are 15 men and 30 women among them. 23 patients reported their olfactory to be decreased, but 22 believe it is normal. 7 PD patients smoke (2 men and 5 women). There were 12 men and 28 women with ET, aged from 22 to 82. 7 patients here reported their olfactory to be decreased, but 3 patients reported the increased olfactory. 30 patients believe it is normal. 7 patients (2 men and 5 women) smoke.

3.1.1. First Subtest

The first subtest aims to determine the olfactory threshold. The average score over this subtest for PD patients was 2.44; the minimal score is (obviously) 0, and the maximal one is 7. The patients with ET showed the average score

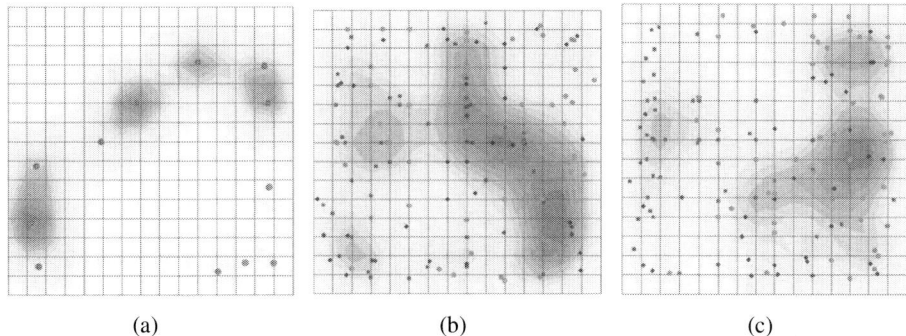

Figure 1. The distribution of PD patients, ET patients and healthy persons in elastic map, over the data of the first subtest (Fig. 1(a)), over the second subtest (Fig. 1(b)) and over the third subtest (Fig. 1(c)).

equal to 3.85, with minimal and maximal figures equal to 0 and 9, respectively. Finally, the corresponding figures observed in control group were 5.10, 0 and 11, respectively.

3.1.2. Second Subtest

The second subtest aims to measure the ability to discriminate: a testee is to recognize two identical smells from three probes. The average score over this subtest in PD group was 8.76, whereas the minimal score was 1, and the maximal one was 13. For ET patients, the average score was 10.00, with minimal and maximal figures equal to 4 and 15, respectively. The control group average score was 11.53, whereas minimal and maximal ones were 4 and 15, respectively.

3.1.3. Third Subtest

The third subtest aims to measure the identification ability of a patient; a patient is to refer the presented smelling stick to an object to be chosen from the set of four items. The patients with PD identified the smell of fish best of all. The worst results in smell identification have been observed for lemon and apple; minimal score observed in this subtest was 0, and the maximal one was 13, with average equal to 6.78.

Table 2. Correlations between the probes at the first subtest of Sniffin' sticks test carried out due to standard protocol, for healthy people, j is the number of probe

	4	5	6	7	8	9
3	1.000**	0.529	0.258	0.200	0.135	0.135
4		0.529	0.258	0.200	0.135	0.135
5			0.488	0.378	0.255	0.255
6				0.775**	0.522	0.522
7					0.674*	0.674*
8						1.000**

The patients with ET exhibited the best recognition of a garlic smell, while lemon smell was the worst in recognition. Minimal score observed in this group was equal to 5, and the maximal one was 14, whereas the average was 10.08. Control group exhibited the best recognition for garlic smell, but the worst one for lemon and liquorice; we provide the detailed discussion of this point further. The minimal score observed in control group was 6, and the maximal one was 16, with the average equal to 11.28.

For PD patients, anosmia was found for 14 persons (31.1 %); hyposmia was observed for 30 persons (66.7 %). One patient (that is 2.2 % of the group) exhibited the score equal to 30 that is the minimal norm threshold. In the group of ET patients, the anosmia was found for 2 persons (5 %), 31 patients (77.5 %) exhibited hyposmia and normal olfactory was observed for 7 persons (17.5 %). In control group, anosmia was found for 3 persons (4.7 %), hyposmia was found for 32 persons (50 %), and normal olfactory was found for 29 persons (45.3 %). All the data were generalized and presented according to the standard protocol, see Table 1.

The groups were tested for distinguishability with Student test, or Mann-Whitney test. The test choice was determined by the normality of the data distribution; that latter has been checked with Shapiro-Wilk test. All these groups distinguish reliably, with the significance level $\alpha = 0.05$.

3.2. Clustering of the Patients Over Sniffin' Sticks Test Data Reveals Some Systematic Bias

Conventional statistics unambiguously approved the distinguishability of the groups of patients with different extrapyramid neurological disorders, when compared over the olfactory records obtained due to Sniffin' sticks test. An implementation of a diagnostic tool based on olfactory function measurements requests for the solution of a dual problem: an identification of a disease type relying on the smell measurements data, solely, regardless the *á priori* knowledge of the disease of a patient.

An unsupervised clustering (or unsupervised classification) is a sounding method to address the problem mentioned above. It answers the question whether the olfactory function records provide a separation of testees into distinct groups, and if it is so, whether the groups comprise the patients with the same disease; of course, the distinguishability of healthy persons is required, also. We have pursued this approach using elastic map technique (Gorban and Zinovyev, 2015, 2010, 2007).

We have checked clustering over the records of all three subtests, individually, see Figs. 1(a) through 1(c). In these figures, control group is shown in green labels, PD patients are shown in red labels, and ET patients are shown in blue labels. No clustering has been observed over the records of the first subtest; indeed, careful examination of Fig. 1(a) unambiguously shows that the subtest fails to distinguish PD patients from ET patients, not speaking about the healthy persons (control group). There are some clusters, meanwhile, they comprise the patients of all types, both sick, and healthy ones. Moreover, the point corresponding to the patients are on the same projection, so that one fail to distinguish them. This indistinguishability may result from equally low scores exhibited by the testees at the first subtest. On the contrary, the second (Fig. 1(b)) and the third (Fig. 1(c)) subtests provided the separation quite effectively.

The distribution of the patients from control group developed over the data provided by the second and the third subtests simultaneously is shown in Fig. 2(a). The second subtest results are shown in pink pentagons, and the third subtest data are shown in violet circles. The key idea standing behind this clustering is a examination of particular independence of these two subtests: since a direct correlation calculation is quite doubtful, for this type of data, we have checked whether the patients spread separately, in different clusters, if clustering is provided over the combined data. Fig. 2(a) explicitly shows that these two

Table 3. Correlations between the probes carried out in the first subtest of Sniffin' sticks test observed in the control group; j is the number of a probe

	2	3	4	5	6	7	8	9	10	11
1	0.488**	0.293*	0.250*	0.152	0.101	0.085	0.048	0.037	0.023	0.016
2		0.600**	0.511**	0.312*	0.207	0.174	0.098	0.075	0.046	0.033
3			0.852**	0.520**	0.345**	0.290*	0.163	0.125	0.077	0.054
4				0.610**	0.404**	0.340**	0.191	0.147	0.091	0.064
5					0.662**	0.558**	0.313*	0.241	0.149	0.104
6						0.842**	0.472**	0.364**	0.224	0.157
7							0.561**	0.432**	0.266*	0.187
8								0.770**	0.475**	0.333**
9									0.617**	0.433**
10										0.701**

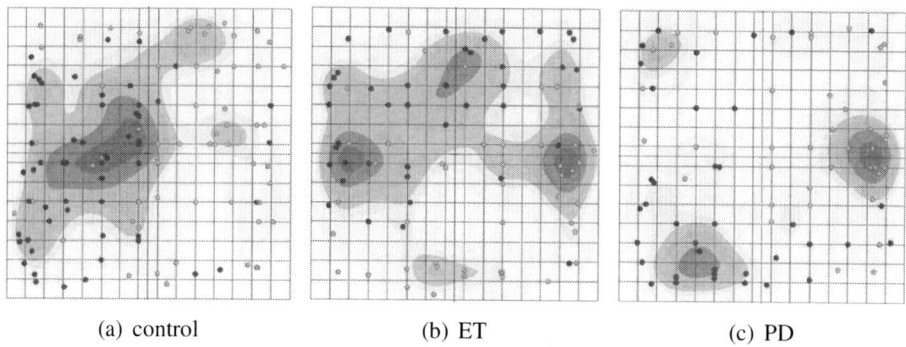

(a) control (b) ET (c) PD

Figure 2. Elastic maps showing the distributions of control group (subfig. 2(a)), ET patients (subfig. 2(b)) and PD patients (subfig. 2(c)), over the data provided by the second and the third subtests.

tests provide rather independent clustering, thus being informative when used separately.

The distributions of PD patients and ET patients over the data of those two subtests are shown in Fig. 2(b) and 2(c), respectively. Again, a differentiation of the subtest data is evident, in these figures, thus approving the feasibility of these data for further comprehensive analysis. Remarkable fact is that the coalescence of the data records from all three subtests annihilates any cluster patterns observed previously.

3.3. Revised Protocol for the First Subtest of Sniffin' Sticks Test to Determine the Absolute Sensitivity Threshold

The results presented in subsec. 3.2 unambiguously confirm the persistence of a systematic error in the results of patients examination provided due to the first subtest of Sniffin' sticks test. The original protocol for this subtest stipulates that a patient perceives a smell, and (s)he is able to detect the threshold of the smell. An adaptation of a smell analyzer of a patient falls beyond the protocol; meanwhile the adaptation takes as long, as 10 seconds to occur.

Table 4. Correlations between the probes carried out in the first subtest of Sniffin' sticks test observed in PD patients group; j is the number of a probe

	2	3	4	5	6	7
1	0.365*	0.243	0.188	0.145	0.098	0.067
2		0.666**	0.515**	0.397**	0.267	0.184
3			0.774**	0.597**	0.401**	0.277
4				0.771**	0.518**	0.358*
5					0.672**	0.464**
6						0.690**

Increased correlation coefficients observed for all couples of the neighbouring probes obtained at the first subtest provide an evidence of this discrepancy. Tables 3, 4 and 7 show the correlation analysis, for the first subtest (j, $1 \leq j \leq 16$ is the number of a probe); table 3 shows the correlations observed in the control group, table 4 shows similar results observed at the PD patients group, and table 7 shows similar results observed at ET patients group. It should be stressed that the test comprises 16 probes, formally. Meanwhile, we have excluded the probes with zero results from the tables. Besides, everywhere further the figures marked with ** sign have the correlation coefficient significance level $\alpha = 0.01$, and those marked with * have the the correlation coefficient significance level $\alpha = 0.05$.

Obviously, the highest correlation coefficients are observed for the couples of probes neighbouring each other, in a series of examinations: $\langle j; j+1 \rangle$, $1 \leq j < 16$. The decay of correlations follows the growth of the "distance" between the probes, and the trend looks quite systematic. Such coordinated variation of the correlation coefficients gives unambiguous evidence on the additional "signal" coming from the testing procedure details. An induction might stand behind this effect: a testee reports on the smell perception, while (s)he is not, indeed. This is the place where olfactory perception psychology manifests.

Table 5. Protocols comparison, see text for details

	ST	UG
$\langle S \rangle$	4.67	8.75
σ	1.92	2.22

We propose a new protocol for the first subtest for the elimination of the discrepancies described above. Actually, the way to avoid the systematic bias in the threshold determination is rather simple: the probes with different concentration of an agents used to examine the perception must be carried out in random order, not in sequential.

To approve the new protocol, we have carried out a pilot testing; that latter was executed with healthy persons, only. It should be stressed that here we tested a new set of testees, in comparison to the experiment described in above. Total number of persons participated at the test was 12, 5 men and 7 women were among them. A verification of the new protocol included two runs of the test; the same testees were invited to run it. At first, the testees ran through the standard protocol examination of the olfactory threshold. Two weeks later, the same testees had been tested following the upgraded protocol. All the testees were healthy people and their daily activities met no restrictions. Thus, the period between these two examinations was long enough to eliminate any recall on the previous survey.

The correlations determined between the different probes obtained in these two examinations are shown in Table 2 and Table 6, correspondingly. Take a note, that Table 2 has no probes #1, #2 and #11 through #16 since these probes yielded zero results. Similarly, Table 6 has no probes #1, #2 and #4, for the same reason.

Tables 2 and 6 bring unambiguous evidence that the effective upgraded protocol eliminates the systemic bias. Table 5 shows the corresponding figures of the average score $\langle S \rangle$ observed due to the standard protocol vs. the upgraded one, and its standard deviation σ, for standard (textsfST) and upgraded () protocols, respectively. The total score increases when determined under the upgraded protocol. Also, we checked the difference between these two examinations with t-test (the data obtained in this experiment meet the normal distribution law), and that latter is reliable, for $p < 0.001$.

Table 6. Correlations between the probes at the first subtest of Sniffin' sticks test carried out due to the upgraded protocol, for healthy people, j is the number of probe

	5	6	7	8	9	10	11	12	13	14	15	16
3	-0.200	0.000	-0.200	0.200	0.258	0.000	0.378	-0.775**	-0.258	-0.258	-0.400	0.447
5		0.447	0.400	0.200	0.258	0.447	0.378	0.258	0.258	0.258	0.200	0.000
6			0.447	0.000	0.192	0.000	0.169	-0.192	-0.192	0.192	0.000	0.000
7				-0.400	0.258	0.000	0.378	-0.258	-0.258	0.258	0.200	0.000
8					-0.258	0.447	0.076	0.258	0.258	-0.258	-0.200	0.447
9						0.192	0.293	-0.333	-0.333	0.111	-0.258	0.192
10							0.169	0.192	0.192	0.192	0.000	0.667*
11								-0.488	-0.488	-0.488	-0.378	0.169
12									0.556	0.111	0.258	-0.192
13										0.556	0.775**	-0.192
14											0.775**	-0.192
15												-0.447

Hence, the impact of the procedure of the data collection on the smell perception is proven. This bias may affect seriously the examination results obtained from PD patients, or ET patients, thus deteriorating both diagnostics, and medical treatment prescriptions. Obviously, this fact must be taken into account when using Sniffin sticks test for the purposes of neurological diseases investigations. Still, additional studies are required to improve the accuracy and some other issues of that technique.

3.4. Modification of the Protocol of the Third Subtest of Sniffin' Sticks Test (Odor Identification)

The third subtest aims to detect so called odor identification. In simple words, a testee smells something and then answers the question what this smell recalls him or her most of all. Only one option could be fixed, finally. The score is

Table 7. Correlations between the probes carried out in the first subtest of Sniffin' sticks test observed in ET patients group; j is the number of a probe

	2	3	4	5	6	7	8	9
1	0.397*	0.331*	0.281	0.187	0.141	0.096	0.037	0.037
2		0.832**	0.707**	0.471**	0.356*	0.243	0.092	0.092
3			0.850**	0.567**	0.427**	0.291	0.111	0.111
4				0.667**	0.503**	0.343*	0.131	0.131
5					0.754**	0.514**	0.196	0.196
6						0.682**	0.260	0.260
7							0.381*	0.381*
8								1.000**

determined according to the sum of the correct answers.

This type of tests belongs to so called attended knowledge tests (see e.g.,, (Schurer et al., 2020; Goodhew et al., 2020; Malim, 2017; McMullen et al., 2016)), similar to spontaneous brand awareness, in ads and marketing (Domazet et al., 2017). The point is that the out-come of such testing severely depends on the fine details of the questioning procedure. In particular, we have found significant biases in the texting results provided by the third subtest of Sniffin' sticks test, when examined both neurological patients, and healthy people.

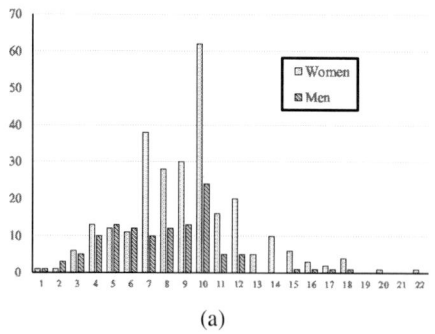
(a)

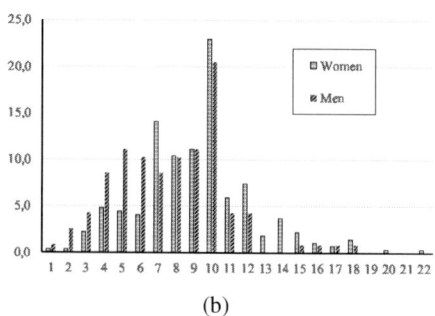
(b)

Figure 3. The distribution of number of recalled smells, by women (red) and men (blue).

3.4.1. How Many Smells Do a Respondent Recall?

Fig. 3 shows the distribution of smells number recalled by respondents; dark gray bars show the numbers of smells recalled by men, and light grey bars shows similar numbers for women. In particular, Fig. 3(a) shows the distribution of the absolute numbers of the smells, and Fig. 3(b) shows the same data expressed in percents. Obviously, some difference is observed between women and men, if the difference is measured in percentage rate. Average number of recalled smells was $7,69 \pm 3,15$ for men and $9,21 \pm 3,25$ for women. We tested these data for normality with Shapiro-Wilk test; the test shows non-normality of the data distribution. Thus, we applied Mann-Whitney test to check whether sexual difference in the number distribution takes place, or not. The men's numbers differ from the women's ones, with $p < 0,001$. Also, χ^2-test approves the distinguishability of the number of smells distributions between men and women, for $p = 0.04$.

Fig. 3 shows an unexpected peak at the smell number equal to 10. It should be stressed that this is an artifact coming from the discrepancy in interviewing technology; see details in subsec. 4.3.

3.4.2. Reference Level: What Smells Do a Respondent Recall?

Studying the features of a normal smell perception starts from the investigation of the number of these latter typically recalled by a respondent (either in a control group, or in the group of sick patients). Next question is the composition of the ensembles of the smells they have recalled.

To answer this question, we have carried out special investigation addressing this problem. To do it, we interviewed students of Krasnoyarsk state medical university and Siberian federal university. The former respondents were the four year students of medicine (general practice), and the latter were the first year students of computer science. The interview was anonymous and to collect the data, each respondent was supplied with special paper questionnaire form. The form has two mandatory fields: age and sex, and ten numbered blank lines to write down the smells they recall. An interview started from the brief story explaining the aim of the research; the story was performed to conspire the real goal of the study. Next the respondents have been instructed to write down their age and sex into the relevant boxes in the form.

As soon, as all the respondents in a room completed to fill out these two mandatory fields, they were instructed to fill the blank lines in their forms with the smells, as they recall it. The instruction was to go on with the filling out, over the opposite side of the form, if the number of smells exceeds the number of blank lines. Time period for the answers was as long, as one minute. Any answering has been aborted upon this time period.

The databases were developed independently, for these two groups of students; later we checked whether these two bases differ or not. No statistical difference between them has been found, so the bases were merged into the common one. The joint database comprises 387 conditionally healthy people; there were 271 women and 116 men in it. The average women age is $21,66 \pm 3,47$ years vs. $21,03 \pm 2,08$ for men. All the conditions during the interviewing were the same, to minimize the impact of under-controlled factors: fresh air, no noise, comfort illumination in auditorium (since they answered in written form).

Figure 4 shows the distribution of the numbers of recalled smells, be women (light grey bars) and by men (dark grey bars). The data are sorted in descending order, according to women's answers. Perfume, petrol and orange were the most frequent items memorized by the respondents. Remarkably, perfume is the leading item to be recalled both in women, and in men audience. However, this item is indeed an aggregated: in reality, the respondents (of both sexes) pointed out a huge variety of the smells which were gathered into *perfume* category. Similar cumulative effect has been observed for *flowers* and *bakery* items. However, *coffee* and *petrol* items were highly specific, both for women and men.

3.5. Comparative Study of Tremor Hyperkinesis of PD Patients vs. ET Patients

The study of tremor included 5 tests; we used *Colibri Neurotech* ™ to measure the tremor. The data were recorded from four locations: on each hand (left and right), and on each forearm (left and right). Five tests have been undertaken to measure the tremor.

The first test measured the tremor in rest.

The second test was recorded when a patient took Romberg maneuver: standing with closed eyes and the arms stretched ahead.

At the third test a patient standing with closed eyes was instructed to touch his/her nose tip with the right hand.

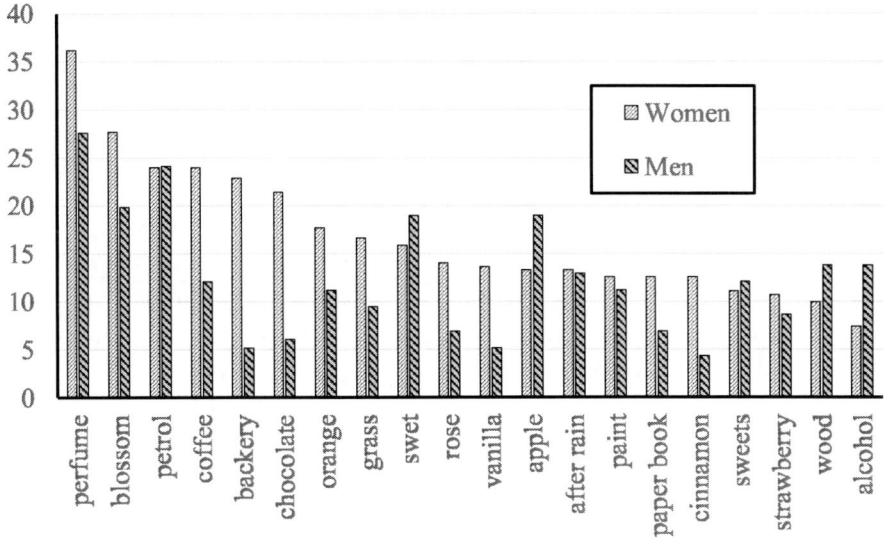

Figure 4. The distribution of number of specific smells recalled by women (light grey bars finely hatched right) and men (dark grey bars coarsely hatched left).

At the fourth test a patient standing with closed eyes was instructed to touch his/her nose tip with the left hand, and finally

The fifth test was executed in a movement, when a patient walked in a room.

Totally 90 persons have been tested for tremor: 30 of them were conditionally healthy, 30 were PD patients, and 30 were ET patients.

Both frequency and amplitude of electromyogram (EMG) were recorded from the left and the right arms of each patient. No statistically significant difference has been detected between the left and the right arms, at the second, the third and the fifth tests, for control group. Similarly, no statistically significant difference has been detected between the left and the right arms, at the first, the second and the fifth tests, for ET patients. This fact may result from the differences in a muscle development, their current condition and a distinction of the subcutaneous fat layer. No difference has been detected, for PD patients. It should be stressed that the average age of PD patients (61 years) along their functional status, one may expect an almost complete lack of any physical training; that is why no predominance of an arm has been detected. Also, one may meet a failure of conventional statistics methods to detect the difference.

Also, we have studied the difference in the recorded data between the groups of patients. Statistically significant difference in the frequency of EMG oscillations recorded at the left arm were found:

- between PD patients and ET patients, for all five tests;
- between control group and ET patients, for the first, the third and the fourth tests;
- between control group and PD patients, for the fifth test.

Also, the statistically significant difference of the data has been found for the records obtained from the sensor located at the right forearm for:
- between PD patients and control group, at the third test;
- between control group and ET patients, at the fourth tests.

Besides, the statistically significant difference in the records obtained from the sensor located at the left forearm has been detected between control group and PS patients.

We analyzed the difference between the groups of patients in terms of EMG amplitudes, as well. At the first test, statistically significant difference for the records from the right hand has been found between PD patients and control group, as well, as between control group and ET patients. Same test yields the difference between ET patients and control group for the records from the sensors located at the right forearm. The records from the sensors located at the left forearm showed significant difference for these two groups at the third and the fifth tests.

The tremor observed for ET patients decreases in rest and when physical activity goes down. On the contrary, PD patients exhibit increase tremor in rest; this type of tremor goes down in a movement or some other physical activities of a patient. These distinctions may stand behind the statistical difference described above. However, a remarkable fact is the lack of the difference when observed for each sensor location. This fact may be an evidence of the variation in the type of tremor, for different patients. It may manifest a failure of the conventional statistics to detect the difference, either.

EMG oscillation frequency seems to be more informative, in comparison to the amplitude of that former: indeed, no one test yielded statistically significant difference between PD patients and ET patients. However, EMG oscillation frequency records reveal the difference between PD patients, and ET patients in all five tests, for the sensors located at the left hand, whereas similar records from the sensors located at the right hand failed to do it. Probably, this fact comes from the strong prevalence of right-handed persons, in a population, so the left hand is both less developed and less controlled.

3.6. Differentiation of PD Patients from ET Patients Provided by Combined Testing of Tremor and Olfactory

We implemented elastic maps to reveal the difference between PD patients and ET patients in olfactory function records. Fig. 5 shows these maps. Subfig. 5(a)

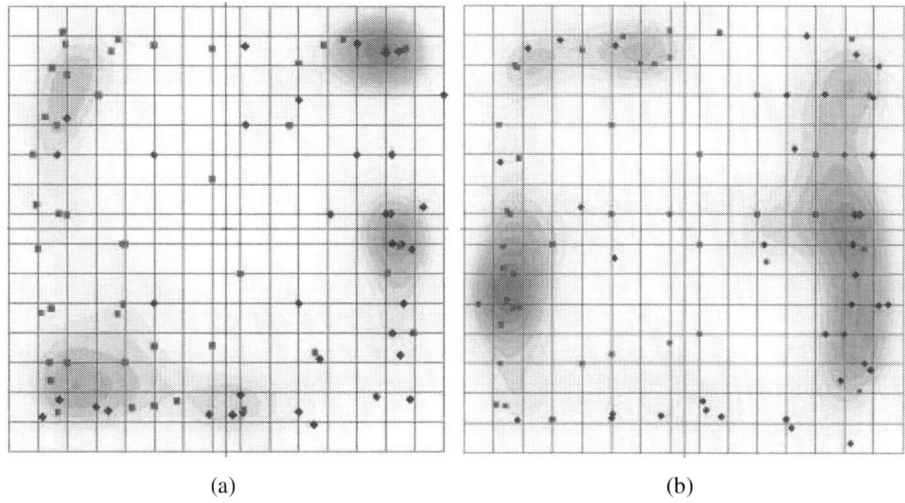

(a)   (b)

Figure 5. Elastic maps showing the distributions of PD patients and ET patients over complete set of olfactory subtests (subfig. 5(a)) and over the records from the second the third subtests (subfig. 5(b)), over the data provided by the second and the third subtests.

shows the elastic maps with PD patients (shown in red squares) and ET patients (shown in blue triangle) distributed over the elastic map implemented for all the records of three subtests.

Both maps show clear separation of PD patients from ET ones. However, there are some patients who escaped clustering. So, we have identified the following groups of the patients:

- those who comprised the clusters (four ones and three ones, respectively), and
- those who escaped from clustering.

Obviously, there are four distinct cluster in Fig. 5(a) and at least three ones in Fig. 5(b). As soon, as the cluster had been identified, they were tested with conventional statistics (t-test, to be exact) against each other, for distinguishability. That latter has been checked for each probe in every subtest. For the case of clustering over all three subtests, statistically significant difference was found for the second and the third probe of the first subtest, only ($p = 0.006$ and $p = 0.023$, respectively). Similarly, the sixth probe of the third subtest exhibit reliable distinguishability with $p = 0.002$. No other probe exhibits the distinguishability. An exclusion of the records of the first subtest from the dataset resulted in occurrence of the statistically significant difference of the clusters:

- over the seventh probe of the second subtest ($p = 0.001$);
- over the total score of the second subtest ($p = 0.029$);
- over the ninth probe and the thirteenth probe of the third subtest ($p = 0.015$ and $p = 0.008$, respectively).

Next, we implemented elastic maps over the data on tremor, only; see Fig. 6. Here PD patients are shown in red squares, and ET patients are shown in blue triangles.

The clusters shown in maps in Fig. 6 comprise both PD patients and ET patients. In other words, rather poor separation of the patients with different diagnosis has been achieved. This failure may result from the excessive tremor data: indeed, tremor records comprise 280 fields, for each patient, in comparison to 52 fields describing the olfactory function. Such excess may deteriorate the signal, keeping in mind the prevalence of the rough data in tremor records. *Rough data* here means they are of all-or-none type; in such capacity, these data do not provide a good discrimination of the objects standing behind.

Hence, we identified the most informative variables in the set of tremor records. There are a number of approaches to figure out such informative variables (see, e.g., (Fukunaga, 1990; Sadovsky, 2006; Shi et al., 2014; Gorban and Zinovyev, 2007)). However, we pursued here the simplest way just through the visual analysis of the histograms of the patients developed over each record field, for tremor data. Indeed, we selected the fields with the histogram mostly close to a normal distribution function, with a single mode, and bell-shaped

All Around the Nose of Parkinsonism and Essential Tremor 121

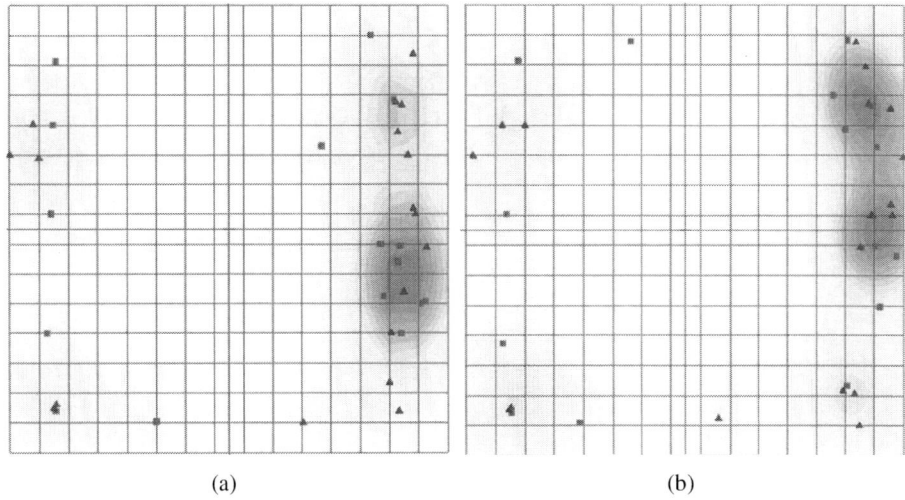

Figure 6. Elastic maps showing the distributions of PD patients vs. ET patients over complete set of tremor records (subfig. 6(a)) and over the combination of tremor records and olfactory testing (subfig. 6(b)).

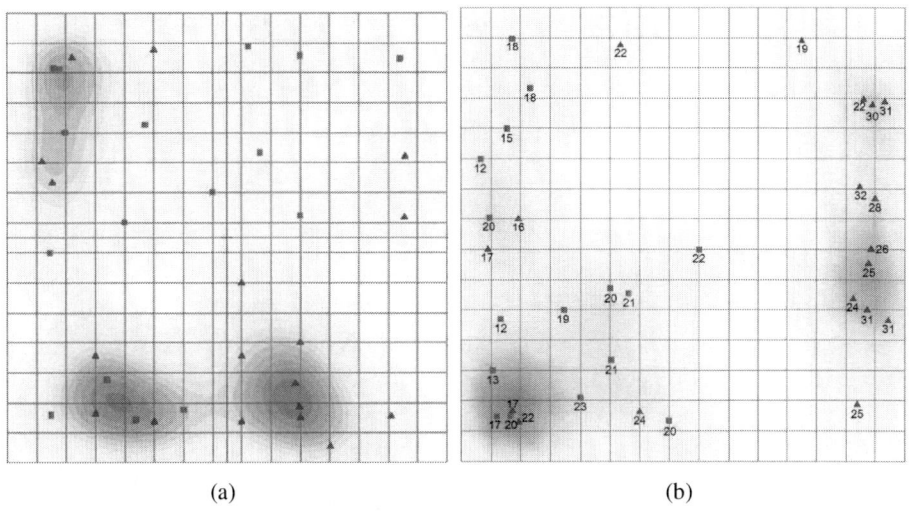

Figure 7. Elastic maps showing the distributions of PD patients vs. ET patients over the selected fields of tremor records (subfig. 7(a)) and over the combination of selected fields of tremor records and olfactory testing (subfig. 7(b)).

form. The selection decreases the number of fields as many, as to 23.

Next, we developed elastic map using the tremor data fields selected previously (see Fig. 7(a)), as well as the map using the combined selected tremor records, and olfactory data (see Fig. 7(b)). Again, red squares label PD patients, and blue triangles label ET patients. It is evident, that the combination of the records (these selected fields of tremor data, and olfactory data) yield much better clustering of the patients, forming three distinct clusters (see Fig. 8). Again, the clusters have been identified through the non-linear statistical technique (that is elastic mapping), however we checked the distinguishability of the clusters due to conventional statistical analysis.

The comparison of clusters over the tremor fields and olfactory probes with conventional statistics revealed that statistically significant difference between the first and the second clusters is observed over the unique variable, that is the sum of scores at the third subtest. The third cluster exhibited statistically significant difference from both the first one, and the second one in tremor data, as well as in olfactory data. Moreover, the angle of a deviation of a limb in kinetic test was the only field in tremor records providing a significant difference (gyroscopic data). Hence, the first and the second clusters are indistinguishable; this fact comes from the composition of these two entities. Indeed, these clusters comprise mainly PD patients, whereas the third cluster comprises ET patients.

The analysis of clusters in terms of olfactory function shows that the third cluster (that is ET patients) exhibits better olfactory condition, in comparison to those comprised in the first and in the second clusters (see Fig. 8). Tremor figures are higher for the patients comprising the third cluster. Thus, it confirms our hypothesis toward the inverse relationship between the tremor expression, and the decrease level of the olfactory function. Also, we hypothesize that the patients comprising the first and the second clusters have worse outcome prognosis for their disease. The fact that significant part of ET patients will meet cognitive and affective complications stands behind this unfavorable prognosis. An explanation is clear: the complications mentioned above follow in a tremor reduction.

Thus, in brief, a combined investigation of tremor and olfactory function of the patients with neurodegenerative diseases brings significant improvement both in diagnostics, and in medical treatment, with better prolonged outcome.

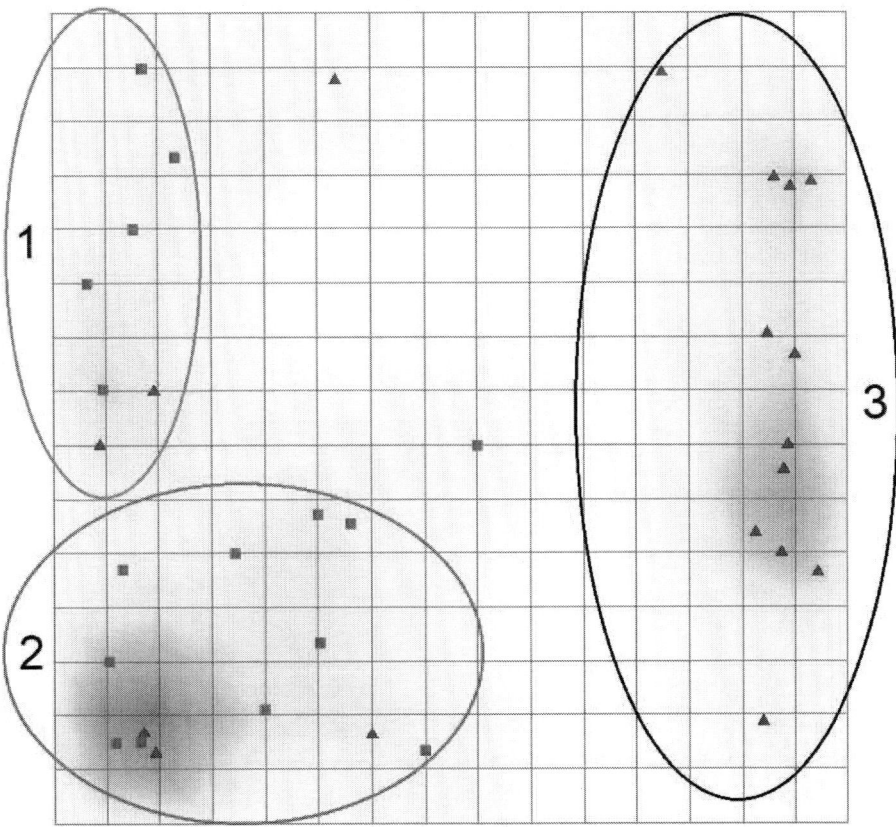

Figure 8. Clustering of PD patients vs. ET patients. Here the clusters are clearly marked with ellipses, in order to clarify the pattern shown in Fig. 7(b); take a note on the total scores observed for the patients (shown in Fig. 7(b)).

4. DISCUSSION

We start the discussion from the tremor/olfactory relations. Later, we change for the discussion of the modification of olfactory testing: this issue includes both Sniffin' sticks test criticism, and provides wider context for the problem discussion.

4.1. Tremor and Olfactory

Olfactory dysfunction is a remarkable fact in PD development appearing few years ahead of the movement disorders. Hyposmia is very common for all patients with PD (Ponomarev and Mazurenko, 2012; Alekseeva et al., 2012; Illarioshkin, 2011; Kostyukova et al., 2016). This fact has a natural explanation: the neurodegeneration starts from the olfactory bulbs of the brain. However, ET has quite different mechanism of the disease; hence, the absence of this symptom for such patients has been reported (Kudrevatykh et al., 2018; Trufanov, 2013).

Thus, olfactory function may play key role in early diagnostics of PD and differentiation of that latter from other type diseases (Chernykova et al., 2015; Fedotova et al., 2015). However, there are quite few reports on olfactory studies with respect to ET, and they are quite contradictory (Titova et al., 2019; Trufanov, 2016; Lacerte et al., 2014; Giorelli et al., 2014).

It should be stressed that decreased olfactory function is the symptom of Alzheimer's disease, also. This pathology has another etiology than PD and ET, being mainly caused by acetylcholine shortage (Voznesenskaya et al., 2011; Kolobov and Storozheva, 2014; Morozova et al., 2014). Combination of tremor data and smell perception data provides a clear and apparent distinction of PD patients from ET ones, as well, as from control group. The results presented above (see subsec. 3.6) bring an evidence of the inverse dependence between tremor level and olfactory function decay; this is the most sounding result of our work.

Indeed, ET patients showed better olfactory function results accompanied by stronger tremor, as compared to PD patients. Few ET patients occupy the cluster comprising PD patients, and the reason of that is the lower olfactory function observed on them. This fact forces to continue their observation in dynamics, keeping in mind that such patients have high chance of PD development in a future. Briefly speaking, the presented results could be implemented for early differential diagnostics of PD vs. ET, as well, as for the improvement of individual therapy course for such patients.

Deep verification of the inverse dependence between olfactory and tremor brings a wider sight on neurological pathology. For example, hot questions here are:

– correlations of the patterns observed over tremor and olfactory (dys)function to cognitive functions of patients, for PD and ET patients;
– same question addressing some other groups of patients with taupathy,

say, Alzheimer's disease.

We believe the implementation of a comprehensive testing methodology based on combination of olfactory function and tremor records for patients with Alzheimer's disease makes a real tool to assess the risk of developing Alzheimer's disease at the preclinical stage. This early diagnostics is of great value here, since this early period of AD development provides a kind of "therapeutic window" to treat it with drugs. Such methodology should imply the following issues:

1) detailed study of smell perception peculiarities through the advanced olfactometry, whether it would be provided by the upgraded Sniffin' sticks test method, or some others;
2) simultaneous testing of patient's cognitive abilities;
3) an implementation of the technique to combine these two types of data to improve sensitivity and specificity of a diagnosis, as well as a systematic assessment of a patient's state.

Verification of the hypothesis on the inverse dependence of smell perception and tremor over the greater set of data is the nearest step in our research. Further studies should address the expansion of the hypothesis for other types of neurodegenerative disorders, first of all, Alzheimer's disease (see also paper by Zalyalova and Bagdanova (2018)).

Also, fine details of the observed inverse dependence patterns should be studied in more detail. The results provided above just prove general trend in interplay between tremor expression and olfactory dysfunction. Even these data show that the pattern seems to be rather complex and versatile. Further investigations in this area may reveal a number of peculiarities in the dynamics of various neurodegenerative diseases.

4.2. Upgrade and Modification of the Methods in Olfactometry

Here we discuss in detail the problems in olfactometry standing behind the modifications and upgrade of Sniffin' sticks test. Of course, there are some other test systems in olfactometry; University of Pennsylvania smell identification test is the most well-known among them. However, we shall not discuss here other olfactory systems, but Sniffin' sticks test. The comparative study of different olfactory systems still awaits researchers.

To begin with, let us list again the failures of the current version of Sniffin' sticks test. Currently effective protocol of an investigation with this test is described in subsec. 2.2. Here we discuss some approaches to adapt the techniques of olfactory dysfunction measurements provided by the standard protocol of Sniffin' sticks test for the purposes of early diagnostics of Parkinson's disease and differentiation of that latter from essential tremor. The approved and standard Sniffin' sticks test is described in detail in papers (Krismer et al., 2017; Lawton et al., 2016; Sorokowska et al., 2015). There are some attempts to apply the test for children examination (Hugh et al., 2015), as well as into the related areas (Caglayan et al., 2016).

So, here are the disadvantages of the standard protocol of the test.

1) Regular (ordered descendingly of the concentration of a smelling agent) exposition of smelling sticks to a testee causes a kind of adaptation and induction in the smell perception: a testee reports on the perception of the smell, while (s)he does not. We believe, induction is the main mechanism of such effect: a person knows (s)he is expected to report on the smell, and tends to report on it.
2) The second subtest is poorly localized, under the currently effective protocol. The names of the subjects to be used to check the smell identification are very uncommon, for persons with Russian mother language. A testee may know nothing on these names, and the answer would be biased through the reflexivity in case of so called *indifferent choice*.
3) All the subtests may not be properly interpreted without the reference list of smells and their circulation rate typical for the given population.

Let now discuss the above mentioned disadvantages in more detail. Ordered (*backward staircase method*) testing of the smell perception threshold bring a serious bias, in the observations. It may result from two processes: the former is adaptation, and the latter is induction. Adaptation may really improve the perception, if a measurement is arranged in ordered way. The induction seems to be more psychological than physiological, however it deteriorates the results. A testee reports on the perception just because (s)he imagine it, with no real sensing of the low concentration smell. Paper (Eluecque et al., 2015) shows that randomization of the probes order at the first subtest yields the figures of the indicators of threshold odor perception significantly different from similar ones obtained under the backward staircase method (original technique);

besides, randomization saves time for testing.

The problem of the third subtest consists in the absence of the reference for evaluation of the smell recognition. In other words, what is the baseline to compare the observed answers on the smell identification? What names/items must be referred as (extremely) rare, and which ones are supposed to be typical? Thus, the question arises whether the list of answers collected from testees represents a normal choice in a population, or it is biased? To resolve the problem, one must know the level of so called *unattended knowledge* of various smells (see further details below).

The first bias reason comes from specific cultural, psychological and linguistics constraints: indeed, the original protocol stipulates that the identification is revealed through the choice of a subject that corresponds most of all to the smell. A testee is provided with a card bearing four words, not the objects (as a picture). Here a great rupture may take place, between the real perception, and the knowledge of the word proposed for recognition.

For example, the words *liquorice* ([lakritza], in Russian), *turpentine* and *anise* ([anis], in Russian) are familiar to a minority of testees. The point is that the original protocol provides these words only. The words are in the Russian vocabulary, while they are at the ultimate periphery of linguistic uses. Clumsy thing is that there are two Russian exactly matching synonyms for these two words: [solod], in Russian and [ukrop], in Russian. These names are very familiar to anybody speaking Russian.

So, briefly speaking, the on-going protocol of the third subtest of Sniffin' sticks test is not linguistically localized. It yields various biases in testee answers, and fall beyond the control of a doctor or a researcher. Some approaches to eliminate the biases are discussed further.

It should be stressed that this failure may result from the cultural divergence of the local residents. The point was that the patients have been asked to indicate the object within a kit presented after the odorous stimulation, that has the peculiar smell, upon the mind of a patient. This is a kind of so called *attended knowledge*, and the reliability of an answer heavily depends on the consistency of a stimulation. In other words, the object used for stimulation must be well known to a recipient; meanwhile, they were not.

Let now focus on Fig. 3; one can see an unexpectedly increased number of respondents reporting on ten smells they have recalled. Indeed, that is an artifact resulting from the technical presentation of the form for answering the recalled smells. Each testee was provided with a blank form and has been instructed to write down all the smells (s)he can recall immediately. The point is that the form looks actually as a table with ten blank lines; the testees were instructed to turn over the form and continue to answer, if they recall more than ten items. Obviously, too many respondents stopped answering upon the completion of these ten lines. Further, we shall use another type of the form, with as many blank lines as 40, just to eliminate the unconscious constraint provided be the improper questionnaire form. We believe, 40 items is enough, since it exceeds approximately twice the maximal number of the reported smell recalls (see Fig. 3). It should be kept in mind that answering must be not longer than a minute.

This artifact does not affect our results, since we aimed to study the diversity of the specific smells recalled by testees, not the number of recalled items, see Fig. 4. In such capacity, we tried to identify the most widely circulated smells in a population, to get the reference for the smells recalled by PD and ET patients (see subsec. 4.3 below).

Still, some essential questions towards the feasibility of the test are not answered. To begin with, we believe the key problem in Sniffin' sticks test arises from the general psychological problem with deep evolutionary and biological roots: no language worldwide has specific ("own" or proper) lexicon to describe smell world (Barkat-Defradas and Motte-Florac, 2016). In simple words, everything related to sense of smell falls beyond (rational) consciousness. Thus, one should understand that any knowledge retrieved from any experiment of testing related to the sense of smell is indirect and must be verified.

From that point of view, the second test looks best of all. The point is that the ability to differentiate something in senses works much better, for human beings, than ability of the direct detection. The second test is based on the differential evaluation and fits this human ability best of all. The third test looks worse from that point of view. First of all, it requires a cultural (and, maybe, ethnic) adaptation: there is no guarantee that people belonging to different races and ethnicities always respond similarly, in reaction on a smell stimulation.

4.3. Unattended Knowledge of Smells: Some Calamities

Let now focus on the results of the smell recall numbers (see subsec. 3.4.1 on page 115).

4.3.1. Reflexivity

Another problem arises from human consciousness resulting in inability to behave randomly. Suppose, we carry out a series of testing where the sticks used in the examination are odorless (or the concentration of a smelling agent is below the perception threshold); the instruction of a test stipulates that the odor is very weak, slightly above the perception threshold. Meanwhile, the task is to separate those sticks into two groups: the former must comprise smelling sticks, and the latter must comprise the odor-free sticks. A naïve expectation is that the testees separate the sticks into almost equal in number sets. In reality, the reflexivity of human consciousness (Lefebvre, 2013) breaks down random behaviour, and the separation yields the figure of the golden ratio. Thus, the first test of Sniffin' sticks test may not be interpreted correctly, unless the impact of two factors described above is implemented into the protocol.

Nonetheless, the second and the third tests have high diagnostics value; doubtlessly, they could be used in medical practice. Moreover, the development of elastic map over a set of carefully collected reference set of healthy people and patients with PD may bring a lot into the early diagnostics and identification of the group at risk; the data shown in Fig. 8 illustrate it unambiguously. Yet, the practical implementation requires more detailed studies. Besides, this approach could be applied for a study of some other neurological diseases, say, essential tremor. We have tried the methodology in analysis of this kind of patients, and have obtained positive results. Meanwhile, the detailed discussion of these issues falls beyond the scope of this chapter.

4.3.2. Unattended Smell Knowledge: Some Approaches to Exclude Uncontrolled Affects

A number of various factors may affect the results of olfactometry. Some of them may be under control of experimentalist, others are out of it. Odor environment, as well, as the subjects surrounding a testee, temperature are among the factors under experimentalist's control. Some factors may be controlled by experimentalist: for example, satiety level may be controlled. A number of factors are semi-controlled: for example, physiological status of a respondent may not be controlled completely. Finally, some factors are out of control: for example, a mood of a respondent, or emotions if they are induced by outer circumstances.

The accentuation of odors in reports may also be associated with the pro-

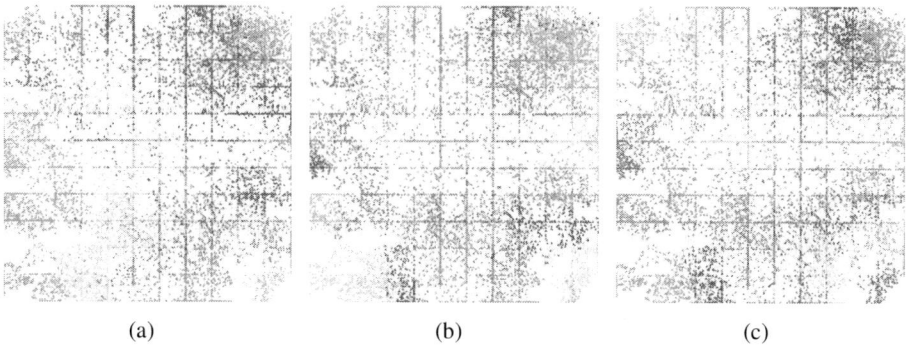

Figure 9. An example of visual task aimed to switch off the under controlled affects of a reasoning on a smell recalling.

fession of a respondent. Thus, a car driver would recall petrol and engine oil odors reliable more often, in comparison to an average frequency of these items appearance in the averages figures determine over a population. Reciprocally, a florist would preferably recall flowers smells; medicians would recall the smell of alcohol or other medical stuff. Again, the absence of a proper lexicon for olfactory sensing makes the problem worse. Even blood tension measurement may be affected by an *á-priori* knowledge (Salvetti et al., 2019).

There are some approaches to decrease the impact of those uncontrolled factors in olfactometry. Here we discuss an option to do it. We tried to use a kind of gag to kill the affects from uncontrolled factors, at least, some of them. The gag is kind of a task specially offered to a respondent to draw his/her out of the core task. We used the following procedure to do it: respondents have been supplied with specially designed form. The face side of form bears a picture, and a respondent has been requested to do some exercise before doing the proper smell reporting. Fig. 10 shows the pattern. The "gag" task was to count all the convex pentagons you might figure out in this picture; this task was as long, as a minute. As soon, as the "gag" task was completed, a respondent was immediately instructed to turn over the form and to fill the blanket located on the other side of the form with the names of the subjects associated with the smells (s)he can recall immediately.

The main goal of the gag task is the concentration of the attention of a respondent on a subject that has nothing to do with real investigation; in such capacity, no matter whether the number of those pentagons is correct, or wrong.

All Around the Nose of Parkinsonism and Essential Tremor 131

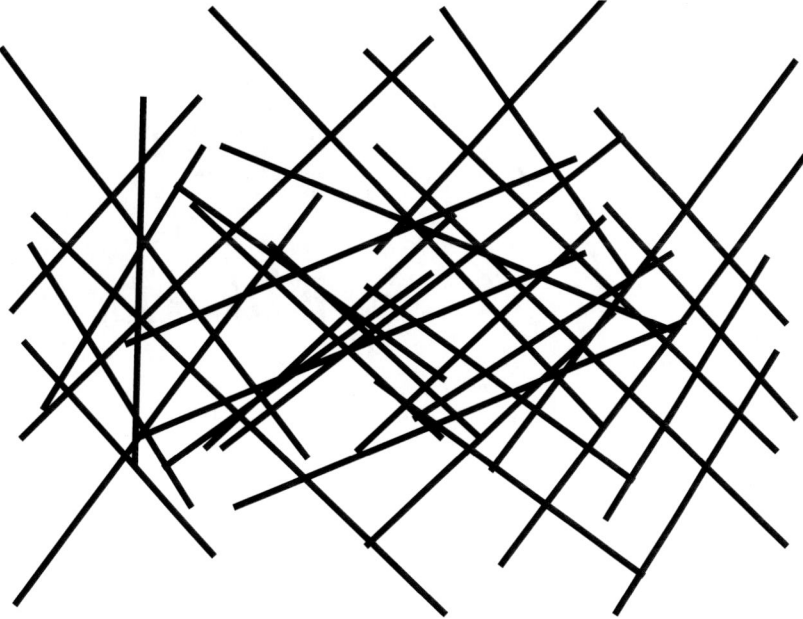

Figure 10. An example of the gag used to avoid under-controlled factors impact in olfactometry of unattended smell recalls.

No one ever checked them, at all.

Another type of stimuli that might be used to divert attention of a respondent from the essential task is shown in Fig. 9. Here the attention deteriorating task was as following. We have generated a series of 24 figures (three of them are shown in Fig. 9); the patterns were obtained in a run of sequential realizations of K-means classifications of $\approx 20\,000$ points located in 63-dimensional Euclidean space. We used the same way of visualization with elastic map technique, as described in subseq. 2.4. We set $K = 24$ (that makes no sense in the original data), so that a great diversity of color labeling of the classes has been obtained. The task was to identify some order in the color appearance; again, no matter the task was.

The idea to divert attention in a study of some physiological or psychological issues is not the new one. Moreover, results of a study may depend on the type of gag used to divert attention. For example, we expect to get different results on smells recalling, if used two different patterns for it; see Fig. 11. Hence,

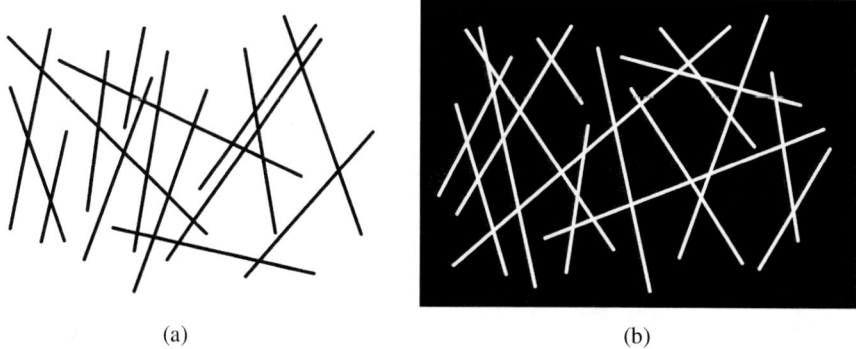

Figure 11. Two versions of (almost the same) gag that may affect the smell recalling results.

an implementation of a gag is a matter of a special study; papers (Bertamini and Kitaoka, 2018; Ashida et al., 2017) consider the patterns causing optical illusion that might be used for this purpose.

It should be stressed that black and white patterns seem to be more preferable, for this type of gag tasks. The point is that flat black and white patterns used for a gag task activate neurophysiological processed ran in the parieto-occipital parts of the cerebral cortex. To be exact, the angular gyrus of the parietal lobe participates in the process of recognition of the depicted elements; that is so called *visuospatial gnosis*. The inferior parietal lobe and the supra-marginal gyrus are involved in the counting process of the lines and intersection points of them. The primary projection zones of cerebral cortex, namely the neurons of the 17-th Brodmann field of the primary visual cortex, respond selectively to certain visual stimuli: on color, on direction and on movement characters of chaotically located lines.

The secondary projection zones of the cerebral cortex comprise the 18-th and the 19-th Brodmann's fields of neurons support the detection of more complex contour elements, such as edges, border lines, intersection angles and their orientation. Associative tertiary projection zones of the cortex comprise the integration level and support the generalization of stimuli; number of elements, their position in space, the interplay of elements in relation to each other are the issues to be generalized.

4.4. Semantic Differential Approach in Olfactometry

One more possible development in olfactometry may come from (related) psychological studies: that is semantic differential determination. In brief, semantic differential consists in the implementation of a kind of *profile* of a respondent, so that the profile (more or less) unambiguously characterizes the respondent.

A *profile* consists of a set of bi-polar scales, where each scale consists of two opposing concepts; the opposition is based on their semantics, not on morphemic issue of word. Simply speaking, there exist two types of antonyms (these are the words with opposite meaning): the former makes the opposition with lexicon, and the latter does it with morphological properties of words. The couple

$$high \iff low$$

is the first type example, whereas the couple

$$cyclone \iff anticyclone$$

is the second type example.

A respondent is asked to evaluate an object through the fitting the scale figure ranging from -2 (one pole, usually strongly negative) to 2 (usually strongly positive) with 0 treated as neutral choice. A set of scales filled by a respondent is expected either to characterise an object, or characterize a person, in dependence on the specific task of a study; see (Hawkins II, 2016; Takahashi, 2018; Themistocleous et al., 2019; Takahashi et al., 2016; Río et al., 2018) for illustrations and details of the method applied to various tasks, including medical ones.

To develop the tool for a research, one must choose the semantically opposing issues, and fix the number of grades. Olfactory is closely related to a taste, and we here illustrate the cultural difference in the opposition using this field of sense. Thus, for people with English as a mother language, a *sweet* taste is opposed by *bitter* taste; for those with Russian mother language the opposition is *salty*; there are some cultures with *acid* opposing the *sweet* taste. One may expect to face similar situation with smells (Detandt et al., 2017; Petrenko and Mitina, 2020). The number of grades also depends on culture and mother language of a respondent. Again, Russian and English speaking people normally may distinguish up to 5 and 12 grades, respectively.

Keeping all these points in mind, we introduce an idea to construct and use in olfactometry specially designed couples of the smells occupying opposite poles in a mind, with due grade scale. Again, the core problem here is the absence of the proper lexicon for smell perception; this fact is claimed to be universal, for all languages worldwide. Thus, the question arises what kind of smells to be considered as opposing ones.

The studies of unattended smell knowledge may address the problem of bi-polar scaling implementation; see subsec. 3.4.1. Indeed, an analysis of smells commonly circulating in cognition of regular population of Russia may improve the choice of the candidates for bi-polarity, for semantic differential implementation in olfactometry.

The grades number is actually a matter of compromise between high accuracy of a detection, and feasibility of a test. Not speaking about the upper estimation of the number of grades culturally predetermined for respondents, one must keep in mind the procedure of examination, as a whole. First of all, the tentative test must be carried out in the most standardized conditions: a number of factors may affect the measurement results, and bias them. For instance, an examination to be carried out in a medical facility may cause a stress, an esurience may affect seriously the results of any smell testing, since that former is deeply related to a smell perception, even in the absence of real food smells (imagination affects). Also, no irritation of a respondent must take place resulting from physiological needs, etc.

Thus, a tentative scheme of olfactometry experiment may be as following: a respondent is provided with a series of verbally expressed bi-polar scales targeted to measure olfactory function. As soon, as experimentalist is sure a respondent clearly understands what kind of polar oppositions (s)he is provided, the respondent is exposed with a smell source being asked to place the odored smell somewhere within the scales. The total score represents the profile of a respondent. Probably, a respondent may experience several odor tests, during the same examination; however, an experimentalist must keep the number of the odors not exceeding, probably, five or six. The constraint comes from adaptation and tiredness of a respondent.

Here we outlined briefly some further developments in methodology of olfactometry; yet, all these issues still await for detailed researches.

Conclusion

Here we present some preliminary results of the combined study of the tremor data records, and olfactory (dys)function observed simultaneously over the patients with Parkinson's disease and essential tremor. These two pathologies are hard to distinguish; previously, a number of attempts had been made to do it over the tremor data, or olfactometry, individually. Neither of the approaches yields a good result; on the contrary, the combination of these two diagnostic tools brings clear and unambiguous distinguishability of the patients suffering from Parkinson's disease, and the patients suffering from essential tremor. Moreover, these two groups both differ from control healthy group, if compared over the combined data records.

The effect of distinguishability requires special tool to reveal it. That is elastic map technique, an up-to-date very powerful and efficient method to analyse multidimensional bulky data through the approximation of them with manifolds of low dimension, and visualize the analysis results.

This advanced technique provided a strong evidence of the validity of the hypothesis on the inverse relationship between tremor and olfactory; simply speaking, the patients with increased tremor exhibit higher smell perception ability, and vice versa. This fact seems to be very important from clinical point of view, since it makes a background for a treatment improvement.

Another important result of this chapter is the valuable protocol improvement, for Sniffin' sticks test. Currently effective protocol yields a number of biases, when applied for clinical or research applications. The first Sniffin' sticks subtest is deteriorated with the excessive regularity in the measurement procedure: that former follows in the growth of adaptation, and psychological influence. Randomization of the measurement procedure results in more reliable and objective results of the smell threshold determination.

The second and the third Sniffin' sticks subtests are not properly grounded, since there is no reference data on smell distinguishability. We proposed a special method to get the reference based on the identification of the smells that recalled by patients, in case of unattended knowledge registration. Our preliminary results support the upgrade of the protocol, since they improve the accuracy and validity of olfactory measurements carried out with Sniffin' sticks test.

One more modification of the effective protocol concerns the second Sniffin' sticks subtest. That latter implies an identification of a specific smell exposed to a testee through the choice of a subject from the set of four ones. Currently, the choice is provided through the written words, not the images of the smelling subjects. The subtest is not localized at least for Russia, since the names of subjects used in the currently effective protocol are not common, for Russian speaking audience.

An improvement of the currently effective protocol of Sniffin' sticks test, its localization and comparison to other tests widely used for olfactory function investigation requires further studies.

REFERENCES

Alekseeva, N. S., S. N. Illarioshkin, T. A. Ponomareva, E. Y. Fedotova, and I. A. Ivanova-Smolenskaya (2012). Smell violations in Parkinson's disease (in Russian). *Neurological journal [Nevrologicheskii zhurnal 17*(1), 10–14.

Altunisik, E. and A. H. Baykan (2019). Comparison of the olfactory bulb volume and the olfactory tract length between patients diagnosed with essential tremor and healthy controls: Findings in favor of neurodegeneration. *Cureus 11*(10), 23 – 34.

Ashida, H., A. Ho, A. Kitaoka, and S. Anstis (2017). The spinner illusion: More dots, more speed? *i-Perception 8*(3), 2041669517707972.

Ault, S. V. (2018). *Understanding Topology: A Practical Introduction*. JHU Press.

Bain, P. (1993). A combined clinical and neurophysiological approach to the study of patients with tremor. *Journal of neurology, neurosurgery, and psychiatry 56*(8), 839.

Barkat-Defradas, M. and E. Motte-Florac (2016). *Words for odours: Language skills and cultural insights*. Cambridge Scholars Publishing.

Benito-Leon, J. and E. D. Louis (2006). Essential tremor: emerging views of a common disorder. *Nature clinical practice Neurology 2*(12), 666–678.

Bertamini, M. and A. Kitaoka (2018). Blindness to curvature and blindness to illusory curvature. *i-Perception 9*(3), 2041669518776986.

Braak, H., K. Del Tredici, H. Bratzke, J. Hamm-Clement, D. Sandmann-Keil, and U. Rüb (2002). Staging of the intracerebral inclusion body pathology associated with idiopathic Parkinson's disease (preclinical and clinical stages). *Journal of neurology 249*(3), iii1–iii5.

Caglayan, H. Z. B., C. Irkec, B. Nazliel, A. A. Gurses, and I. Capraz (2016). Olfactory functioning in early multiple sclerosis: Sniffin'sticks test study. *Neuropsychiatric disease and treatment 12*, 2143.

Chaudhuri, K. R., D. G. Healy, and A. H. Schapira (2006). Non-motor symptoms of Parkinson's disease: diagnosis and management. *The Lancet Neurology 5*(3), 235–245.

Chernykova, I. V., Z. A. Goncharova, K. I. Khadzieva, and E. A. Rabadanova (2015). Clinical predictors of Parkinson's disease (in Russian). *Kuban Scientific Medical Bulletin 152*(3), 134–139.

Chunling, W. and X. Zheng (2016). Review on clinical update of essential tremor. *Neurological Sciences 37*(4), 495–502.

Detandt, S., C. Leys, and A. Bazan (2017). A french translation of the pleasure arousal dominance (pad) semantic differential scale for the measure of affect and drive. *Psychologica Belgica 57*(1), 17.

Domazet, I., I. Dokić, and O. Milovanov (2017). The influence of advertising media on brand awareness. *Management Science 23*, 13–22.

Dorsey, E., T. Sherer, M. S. Okun, and B. R. Bloem (2018). The emerging evidence of the Parkinson pandemic. *Journal of Parkinson's disease 8*(s1), S3–S8.

Eluecque, H., D. T. Nguyen, and R. Jankowski (2015). Influence of random answers on interpretation of the Sniffin'stick identification test in nasal polyposis. *European annals of otorhinolaryngology, head and neck diseases 132*(1), 13–17.

Fahad, A., N. Alshatri, Z. Tari, A. Alamri, I. Khalil, A. Y. Zomaya, S. Foufou, and A. Bouras (2014). A survey of clustering algorithms for big data: Taxonomy and empirical analysis. *IEEE transactions on emerging topics in computing 2*(3), 267–279.

Fedorova, N. V. (2016). Parkinson's disease: Diagnosis and treatment (in Russian). *Contemporary therapy in psychiatry and neurology* (1), 13–17.

Fedotova, E. Y., A. O. Chechetkin, N. Y. Abramycheva, L. A. Chigaleychik, B. K. Baziyan, T. A. Ponomareva, N. S. Alexeeva, P. A. Fedin, M. A. Kravchenko, Y. Y. Varakin, I. A. Ivanova-Smolenskaya, and S. N. Illarioshkin (2015). Identification of people at the latent stage of Parkinson's disease (the PARKINLAR study): first results and an optimization of the algorithm. *S.S. Korsakov Journal of Neurology and Psychiatry = Zhurnal nevrologii i psikhiatrii imeni S.S. Korsakova 115*(6), 4–11.

Fukunaga, K. (1990). *Introduction to statistical pattern recognition.* London: Academic Press.

Fullard, M. E., J. F. Morley, and J. E. Duda (2017). Olfactory dysfunction as an early biomarker in Parkinson's disease. *Neuroscience bulletin 33*(5), 515–525.

Giorelli, M., J. Bagnoli, L. Consiglio, M. Lopane, G. B. Zimatore, D. Zizza, and P. Difazio (2014). Do non-motor symptoms in Parkinson's disease differ from essential tremor before initial diagnosis? A clinical and scintigraphic study. *Parkinsonism & Related Disorders 20*(1), 17–21.

Goodhew, S. C., A. Dawel, M. Edwards, et al. (2020). Standardizing measurement in psychological studies: On why one second has different value in a sprint versus a marathon. *Behavior Research Methods 52*(4), 1156–1172.

Gorban, A. N. and A. Zinovyev (2010). Principal manifolds and graphs in practice: From molecular biology to dynamical systems. *International Journal of Neural Systems 20*(03), 219–232. PMID: 20556849.

Gorban, A. N. and A. Y. Zinovyev (2007). Principal manifolds for data visualisation and dimension reduction. In A. N. Gorban, B. Kégl, D. Wünsch, and A. Y. Zinovyev (Eds.), *Lecture Notes in Computational Science and Engineering* (2nd ed.), Volume 58, pp. 153–176. Berlin – Heidelberg – New York: Springer.

Gorban, A. N. and A. Y. Zinovyev (2015). Fast and user-friendly non-linear principal manifold learning by method of elastic maps. In *2015 IEEE International Conference on Data Science and Advanced Analytics, DSAA 2015, Campus des Cordeliers, Paris, France, October 19-21, 2015*, pp. 1–9.

Haldane, D. and M. Kosterlitz (2016). Of topology and low-dimensionality. *Nature Physics 12*(11), 987.

Halim, Z. and J. H. Khattak (2019). Density-based clustering of big probabilistic graphs. *Evolving systems 10*(3), 333–350.

Hawkins II, R. C. (2016). Weight bias internalization: Semantic differential measurement and treatment implications. *Psychology 6*(12), 748–754.

Hugh, S. C., J. Siu, T. Hummel, V. Forte, P. Campisi, B. C. Papsin, and E. J. Propst (2015). Olfactory testing in children using objective tools: comparison of Sniffin'sticks and university of Pennsylvania smell identification test (UPSIT). *Journal of Otolaryngology-Head & Neck Surgery 44*(1), 10.

Illarioshkin, S. N. (2011). Parkinson's disease course and approaches to early diagnosis. Parkinson's disease and movement disorders. Manual for practical medicians; II Natl. congress (in Russian).

Ivanova, E. O., P. A. Fedin, A. G. Brutyan, I. A. Ivanova-Smolenskaya, and S. N. Illarioshkin (2013). Clinical and electrophysiological analysis of tremor in patient s with essential tremor and Parkinson's disease (in Russian). *Neurological journal [Nevrologicheskii zhurnal] 18*(5), 21–26.

Koçak, T., A. Altundağ, and T. Hummel (2020). Clinical assessment of olfactory disorders. In *All Around the Nose*, pp. 109–112. Springer.

Kolobov, V. V. and Z. I. Storozheva (2014). Modern pharmacological models of Alzheimer's disease (in Russian). *Annals of Clinical and Experimental Neurology = Annaly klinicheskoy i eksperimentalnoy nevrologii 8*(3), 28–44.

Kostyukova, E. S., V. M. Alifirova, N. G. Zhukova, V. A. Petrov, Y. S. Mironova, A. V. Latypova, M. A. Nikitina, M. A. Titova, A. V. Tyakht, Y. B. Dorofeeva, I. V. Saltykova, and A. E. Sazonov (2016). Olfactory dysfunction and modification in microbiota as early non-motor manifestations of Parkinsons disease (in Russian). *Bulletin of Siberian medicine 15*(5), 66–74.

Krismer, F., B. Pinter, C. Mueller, P. Mahlknecht, M. Nocker, E. Reiter, A. Djamshidian-Tehrani, S. Boesch, G. Wenning, C. Scherfler, et al. (2017). Sniffing the diagnosis: olfactory testing in neurodegenerative parkinsonism. *Parkinsonism & related disorders 35*, 36–41.

Kudrevatykh, A. V., M. D. Didur, T. V. Sergeev, D. S. Bug, and I. V. Milyukhina (2018). Non-motor symptoms and quality of life in patients with essential tremor, Parkinson's disease and the combination of essential tremor and Parkinson's disease. *Academic Journal of Medicine 18*(2), 63–71.

Lacerte, A., S. Chouinard, N. Jodoin, G. Bernard, G. A. Rouleau, and M. Panisset (2014). Increased prevalence of non-motor symptoms in essential tremor. *Tremor and other hyperkinetic movements 4*.

Lawton, M., M. T. Hu, F. Baig, C. Ruffmann, E. Barron, D. M. Swallow, N. Malek, K. A. Grosset, N. Bajaj, R. A. Barker, et al. (2016). Equating scores of the university of Pennsylvania smell identification test and sniffin' sticks test in patients with Parkinson's disease. *Parkinsonism & related disorders 33*, 96–101.

Lefebvre, V. A. (2013). *Algebra of conscience*, Volume 30. Springer Science & Business Media.

Levin, O. S., D. V. Artemyev, E. V. Bril, and T. K. Kulua (2017). Parkinson's disease: modern approaches to diagnosis and treatment (in Russian). *Practical medicine 1*(102), 45–51.

Levin, O. S. and V. K. Datieva (2014). Tremor in Parkinson's disease: features in phenomenology and treatment (in Russian). *Contemporary therapy in psychiatry and neurology* (3), 14–19.

Litvinenko, I. V., M. M. Odinak, A. V. Shatova, and O. S. Sologub (2007). Structure of cognitive impairment in different stages of Parkinson's disease (in Russian). *Vestnik voenno-meditzinskoj akademii 3*, 43–49.

Louis, E. D. and J. J. Ferreira (2010). How common is the most common adult movement disorder? Update on the worldwide prevalence of essential tremor. *Movement Disorders 25*(5), 534–541.

Mahlknecht, P., R. Pechlaner, S. Boesveldt, D. Volc, B. Pinter, E. Reiter, C. Müller, F. Krismer, H. W. Berendse, J. J. van Hilten, et al. (2016). Optimizing odor identification testing as quick and accurate diagnostic tool for Parkinson's disease. *Movement Disorders 31*(9), 1408–1413.

Malim, T. (2017). *Introductory psychology*. Macmillan International Higher Education.

Mansur, P. H. G., L. K. P. Cury, A. O. Andrade, A. A. Pereira, G. A. A. Miotto, A. B. Soares, and E. L. Naves (2007). A review on techniques for tremor recording and quantification. *Critical Review^{TM} in Biomedical Engineering 35*(5), 346 – 362.

Masala, C., L. Saba, M. P. Cecchini, P. Solla, and F. Loy (2017). Olfactory function and age: a Sniffin'sticks extended test study performed in Sardinia. *Chemosensory Perception 11*, 19–26.

McMullen, J., M. M. Hannula-Sormunen, E. Laakkonen, and E. Lehtinen (2016). Spontaneous focusing on quantitative relations as a predictor of the development of rational number conceptual knowledge. *Journal of Educational Psychology 108*(6), 857.

Milanov, I. (2007). Clinical and electromyographic characteristics of tremor in patients with generalized anxiety disorder. *Electromyography and clinical neurophysiology 47*(1), 3–9.

Mittal, M., L. M. Goyal, D. J. Hemanth, and J. K. Sethi (2019). Clustering approaches for high-dimensional databases: A review. *Wiley Interdisciplinary Reviews: Data Mining and Knowledge Discovery 9*(3), e1300.

Miwa, T., K. Ikeda, T. Ishibashi, M. Kobayashi, K. Kondo, Y. Matsuwaki, T. Ogawa, H. Shiga, M. Suzuki, K. Tsuzuki, et al. (2019). Clinical practice guidelines for the management of olfactory dysfunction — secondary publication. *Auris Nasus Larynx 46*(5), 653–662.

Morley, J. F., A. Cohen, L. Silveira-Moriyama, A. J. Lees, D. R. Williams, R. Katzenschlager, C. Hawkes, J. P. Shtraks, D. Weintraub, R. L. Doty, et al. (2018). Optimizing olfactory testing for the diagnosis of Parkinson's disease: item analysis of the university of Pennsylvania smell identification test. *npj Parkinson's Disease 4*(1), 1–7.

Morozova, S. V., D. M. Savvateeva, and E. I. Petrova (2014). Olfactory disorders in patients with neurodegenerative diseases (in Russian). *The Neurological Journal 19*(1), 4–8.

Nielsen, T., M. B. Jensen, E. Stenager, and A. D. Andersen (2018). The use of olfactory testing when diagnosing Parkinson's disease — a systematic review. *Danish Medical Journal 65*(5), A5481.

Oh, E. S., J.-M. Kim, Y. E. Kim, J. Y. Yun, J. S. Kim, S. E. Kim, S. B. Lee, J. J. Lee, J. H. Park, T. H. Kim, et al. (2014). The prevalence of essential tremor in elderly Koreans. *Journal of Korean Medical Science 29*(12), 1694–1698.

Oppo, V., M. Melis, M. Melis, I. Tomassini Barbarossa, and G. Cossu (2020). "smelling and tasting" Parkinson's disease: Using senses to improve the knowledge of the disease. *Frontiers in Aging Neuroscience 12*, 43.

Petrenko, V. and O. Mitina (2020). The fairytale semantic differential technique: A cross-cultural application. *Behavioral Sciences 10*(7), 112.

Ponomarev, V. V. and E. V. Mazurenko (2012). Diagnostics of Parkionson's disease at early stage (in Russian). *Medical news [Meditzinskie novosti]* (1), 13–16.

Puschmann, A. and Z. K. Wszolek (2011). Diagnosis and treatment of common forms of tremor. *Seminars in neurology 31*(1), 065–077.

Río, C. J., N. F. Robaina, and J. L. Lucas (2018). Using the semantic differential technique to assess stereotypes toward individuals with disabilities: The relevance of warmth and competence. *Universitas Psychologica 17*(4), 1–12.

Sadovsky, M. G. (2006). Information capacity of nucleotide sequences and its applications. *Bulletin of Mathematical Biology 68*(4), 785–806.

Sakai, K. (2013). *Geometric aspects of general topology*. Springer.

Salvetti, M., A. Paini, C. Aggiusti, F. Bertacchini, D. Stassaldi, S. Capellini, C. De Ciuceis, D. Rizzoni, R. Gatta, E. Agabiti Rosei, et al. (2019). Unattended versus attended blood pressure measurement: relationship with preclinical organ damage. *Hypertension 73*(3), 736–742.

Schurer, T., B. Opitz, and T. Schubert (2020). Working memory capacity but not prior knowledge impact on readers' attention and text comprehension. In *Frontiers in Education*, Volume 5, pp. 26. Frontiers.

Seijo-Martinez, M., M. C. del Rio, J. R. R. Alvarez, R. S. Prado, E. T. Salgado, J. P. Esquete, and M. J. Sobrido-Gomez (2013). Prevalence of essential tremor on Arosa island, Spain: a community-based, door-to-door survey. *Tremor and Other Hyperkinetic Movements 3*, tre–03–192–4299–1.

Shi, Y., A. N. Gorban, and T. Y. Yang (2014). Is it possible to predict long-term success with k-NN? Case study of four market indices (ftse100, dax, hangseng, nasdaq). *J. Phys.: Conf. Ser. 490*, 012082.

Sorokowska, A., E. Albrecht, A. Haehner, and T. Hummel (2015). Extended version of the "Sniffin'sticks" identification test: Test–retest reliability and validity. *Journal of neuroscience methods 243*, 111–114.

Steinley, D. (2010). Stability analysis in k-means clustering. *British Journal of Mathematical and Statistical Psychology 61*(2), 255–273.

Sui, X., C. Zhou, J. Li, L. Chen, X. Yang, and F. Li (2019). Hyposmia as a predictive marker of Parkinson's disease: a systematic review and meta-analysis. *BioMed Research International 2019*, 3753786.

Takahashi, H., M. Ban, and M. Asada (2016). Semantic differential scale method can reveal multi-dimensional aspects of mind perception. *Frontiers in psychology 7*, 1717.

Takahashi, J. (2018). Affective impressions of various disabilities using the semantic differential method. *International Journal of Humanities and Social Science 8*(8), 161–68.

Themistocleous, C., A. Pagiaslis, A. Smith, and C. Wagner (2019). A comparison of scale attributes between interval-valued and semantic differential scales. *International Journal of Market Research 61*(4), 394–407.

Titova, N. V., Y. N. Bezdolny, I. V. Shtuchny, and D. A. Sibetsky (2019). Tremor in Parkinsons disease and essential tremor: practical aspects of differential diagnosis (in Russian). *Meditsinskiy sovet = Medical Council* (9), 46–54.

Trufanov, E. A. (2013). Differential diagnosis and prognosis of Parkinson's disease and essential tremor (in Russian). *Medical Herald of the South of Russia* (1), 22–44.

Trufanov, E. A. (2016). Essential tremor: standards for the diagnosis and treatment (in Russian). *East European Journal of Parkinson's Disease and Movement Disorders 2*(1), 03–11.

Voznesenskaya, A. E., M. A. Klyuchnikova, V. V. Rodionova, and E. I. Voznesenskaya (2011). Olfactory dysfunction in neurodegenerative diseases (in Russian). *Sensor systems = Sensornye sistemy 25*(1), 17–32.

Wang, J. (2012). *Geometric structure of high-dimensional data and dimensionality reduction*. Springer.

White, T. L., A. F. Sadikot, and J. Djordjevic (2016). Metacognitive knowledge of olfactory dysfunction in Parkinson's disease. *Brain and cognition 104*, 1–6.

Wu, L., N. Mu, F. Yang, J. Zang, and J. Zheng (2016). A study of the non-motor symptoms in early Parkinson's disease with olfactory deficits. *Eur Rev Med Pharmacol Sci 20*(18), 3857–3862.

Xu, R. and D. Wunsch (2005). Survey of clustering algorithms. *IEEE Transactions on neural networks 16*(3), 645–678.

Zalyalova, Z. A. (2011). Tremor phenotypes of Parkinson's disease (in Russian). Parkinson's disease and movement disorders. Manual for practical medicians; II Natl. congress (in Russian).

Zalyalova, Z. A. and N. I. Bagdanova (2018). Premotor stage of Parkinsons disease: From hypotheses and theories to clinical practice (in Russian). *Neurological Bulletin 50*(3), 63–68.

INDEX

A

amyloid, viii, 3, 9, 17, 22, 24, 29, 40, 42, 43, 44, 45, 46, 47, 50, 51, 52, 54, 55, 56, 59, 60, 61, 62, 63, 64, 65, 66, 67, 68, 69, 70, 71
amyloid clearance, 54
amyloid plaques, 46, 54, 64, 65
amyloid protein precursor, viii, 40, 42, 43, 44, 45, 51, 54, 59, 64, 67, 69
amyloido-genic metabolism, 51
amyloidosis, 50, 65
amyotrophic lateral sclerosis, 6, 22, 32, 33, 37, 90
animals, viii, 39, 52, 53
anxiety, 53, 142
apoptosis, 13, 23, 26, 28, 29, 30, 31, 32, 37, 49
astrocytes, 5, 16, 30, 33, 35, 46, 49, 50, 51, 63, 68, 81
atherosclerosis, 26, 41, 56, 68
atrophy, viii, 39, 53, 59
autophagy, 9, 11, 14, 26, 27, 28, 30, 34, 35, 37

B

blood, 15, 16, 47, 50, 51, 52, 56, 57, 58, 59, 61, 62, 63, 64, 65, 69, 70, 75, 79, 131, 143
blood-brain barrier, 16, 50, 51, 52, 62, 63, 64, 65, 75, 79
brain, v, viii, ix, 5, 6, 8, 16, 18, 20, 24, 29, 32, 34, 37, 39, 40, 41, 42, 43, 44, 45, 46, 48, 49, 50, 51, 52, 53, 54, 55, 57, 58, 59, 60, 61, 62, 63, 64, 65, 66, 67, 68, 69, 70, 73, 74, 75, 77, 78, 80, 81, 82, 83, 84, 85, 86, 87, 90, 91, 92, 125, 145
brain atrophy, viii, 39, 52, 53, 54, 57
brain hemispheres, 53
brain injury, v, viii, ix, 39, 45, 48, 50, 64, 65, 68, 70, 73, 77, 78, 80, 83, 84, 85, 87
brain ischemia, v, ix, 39, 40, 41, 42, 43, 44, 49, 51, 52, 53, 54, 55, 60, 61, 65, 66, 67, 69
brain parenchyma, 46, 81
brain tissue, 41, 50, 51, 55

Index

C

CA1 and CA3 areas, 55
CA1 area, viii, 39, 42, 49, 67
CA1 neurons, 47
CA3 area, 43, 49, 55, 67
CA3 region, 43, 48
cellular homeostasis, v, 1, 2
central nervous system, viii, 2, 4, 84, 87, 90
cerebral amyloid angiopathy, 45, 50, 69
cerebral cortex, viii, 39, 133
cerebral ischemia, 43, 47, 56, 58, 59, 60, 62, 63, 64, 70, 78
clinical outcome, 47
clustering, 97, 100, 106, 110, 111, 120, 121, 123, 124, 138, 140, 142, 144, 145
cognitive deficit, 53, 68
corpus callosum, 46, 52
cortex, 20, 44, 46, 47, 49, 54, 57, 66, 67, 69, 91, 92, 133

D

death, ix, 4, 6, 7, 8, 13, 15, 17, 18, 20, 26, 27, 31, 34, 46, 47, 48, 49, 51, 54, 55, 61, 73, 74, 76, 77, 78, 80, 82, 83
death of neurons, 54, 55
dementia, vii, viii, 19, 39, 40, 41, 53, 54, 55, 58, 59, 60, 61, 62, 63, 66, 67, 68, 69
differential diagnosis, 97, 99
DNA damage, 6, 12, 15, 17, 27

E

elastic map, 97, 103, 104, 106, 108, 110, 120, 121, 123, 130, 132, 136, 139
endoplasmic reticulum (ER), viii, 2, 3, 5, 9, 10, 11, 15, 18, 19, 23, 24, 26, 27, 31, 32, 33, 36, 37
endoplasmic reticulum stress, 2, 10, 23, 26, 27, 31, 32, 33, 36
energy crisis, 2, 4, 21, 23
epidemiology, 74, 82, 84, 86, 87
ER stress associated degradation (ERAD), 3, 9
essential tremor, vi, vii, x, 95, 97, 98, 100, 102, 104, 106, 107, 108, 110, 112, 114, 116, 118, 120, 122, 124, 126, 127, 128, 130, 132, 134, 136, 138, 139, 140, 141, 142, 143, 144
experimental ischemia, 46, 53
extracellular space, viii, 16, 40, 46, 54

F

folding proteins, viii, 40
functional impairment, 10, 74, 81

G

gene(s), vii, viii, 4, 7, 10, 14, 15, 17, 19, 20, 33, 40, 42, 43, 44, 45, 47, 48, 54, 55, 61, 66, 67
generation plaques, 55
genomic, 41, 67, 70
genotype, v, ix, 39, 40, 41, 54
glial cell, vii, viii, 2, 16, 18, 21, 25, 33, 52, 77

H

healing, 51, 78
healthcare system, 40, 74
hippocampus, viii, 18, 39, 42, 43, 46, 47, 48, 49, 51, 53, 54, 55, 59, 61, 63, 65, 67, 68, 70
human(s), 25, 26, 27, 28, 29, 31, 32, 40, 41, 47, 52, 60, 64, 68, 70, 71, 82, 129, 130
hydrocephalus, 53

I

inflammatory factors, 50, 51
injury, iv, vii, ix, 9, 24, 27, 51, 52, 53, 58, 61, 66, 74, 75, 76, 78, 79, 80, 82, 83, 84, 86, 87
interleukin-1β, 51
ischemia, viii, 6, 24, 39, 42, 43, 44, 45, 46, 47, 48, 49, 50, 51, 52, 53, 54, 55, 56, 58, 59, 61, 62, 63, 64, 65, 66, 67, 68, 69, 70, 82, 87, 91
ischemia episode, 51
ischemia-reperfusion, viii, 24, 39, 45, 48, 50, 65, 70
ischemic brain, viii, 40, 41, 46, 47, 48, 51, 53, 54, 55, 60, 61, 64, 65, 66, 67, 68, 69
ischemic brain injury, 53, 54, 55, 60, 61, 64, 65, 66, 68
ischemic episode, 47, 50
ischemic injury, 44, 51, 59
ischemic stroke, 40, 41, 53, 55, 56, 57, 61, 62, 67, 83

L

lateral ventricles, 46
leukocytes, 51, 79
lymphocytes, 14, 52

M

macrophages, 28, 51, 59, 61, 79
mechanism, 12, 28, 32, 34, 37, 46, 48, 125, 127
medial temporal cortex, 44, 54
memory deficits, 53

hyperphosphorylated tau protein, 48, 49
hyperphosphorylation, 17, 49, 58, 70

microglia, 35, 49, 50, 51, 57, 59, 68, 79, 81, 84, 85
microglial cells, 16
microvessels, 50
monocytes, 51, 59, 61, 79
motor hyperactivity, 53

N

neural network, 51, 145
neurodegeneration, 1, iii, vii, viii, x, 6, 15, 21, 27, 29, 32, 36, 37, 38, 40, 46, 50, 52, 54, 55, 58, 66, 69, 82, 83, 87, 95, 97, 125, 137
neurodegenerative diseases, viii, 2, 4, 5, 8, 11, 14, 17, 21, 24, 25, 26, 31, 33, 38, 99, 123, 126, 142, 144
neurofibrillary tangle(s), 17, 48, 49, 55, 56
neurofibrillary tangle-like, 48, 49
neuroglial cells, 47, 51
neuroinflammation, viii, 39, 53, 57, 68, 79, 83, 86, 88
neuroinflammatory response, 50, 52
neuronal death, 6, 9, 17, 18, 19, 21, 34, 35, 46, 48, 52, 55, 60, 65, 81, 82
neuronal pathology, 50
neuronal survival, 46, 48
neurons, 4, 6, 7, 15, 16, 17, 18, 20, 22, 25, 27, 31, 32, 46, 47, 49, 50, 53, 54, 77, 78, 81, 83, 84, 87, 133
neuropathology, 40, 41, 49, 54, 55, 83
neutrophils, 51, 79
nitric oxide, v, vii, 1, 2, 5, 6, 8, 10, 11, 12, 22, 23, 25, 26, 27, 28, 29, 30, 31, 32, 33, 34, 35, 36, 38, 80, 85
nitric oxide synthase, 2, 25, 27, 28, 29, 33, 80
nitrosative stress, 5, 33

O

olfactory, vii, x, 95, 97, 98, 99, 100, 101, 102, 107, 109, 110, 113, 120, 121, 122, 123, 124, 125, 126, 127, 131, 134, 135, 136, 137, 139, 140, 142, 144, 145
oligodendrocytes, 49, 59, 85
oxidative stress, v, ix, 5, 6, 13, 16, 18, 20, 22, 24, 29, 35, 36, 73, 74, 76, 80, 81, 82, 85
oxidative/nitrosative stress,, 6

P

paired helical filaments, 48, 49
patients, vii, x, 18, 19, 26, 28, 41, 47, 53, 56, 57, 61, 62, 95, 97, 98, 99, 100, 101, 103, 107, 108, 109, 110, 111, 112, 114, 115, 116, 117, 118, 119, 120, 121, 122, 123, 124, 125, 126, 128, 129, 130, 136, 137, 141, 142
phenotype, v, ix, 39, 40, 41, 54, 66, 67
platelets, 50
post-ischemia, viii, 39, 42, 43, 44, 45, 46, 47, 49, 51, 52, 53, 54, 55
post-ischemic brain(s), viii, 40, 41, 42, 46, 47, 49, 50, 51, 54
post-ischemic neuropathology, 53
presenilin 1, viii, 40, 42, 43, 44, 45, 54, 61
presenilin 2, viii, 40, 42, 43, 44, 45, 54, 67
presnilin 1, 42, 43, 44
prognosis, 97, 123, 144
proteasome machinery, 11
protein, vii, viii, 1, 2, 3, 4, 5, 7, 8, 10, 11, 14, 18, 20, 21, 22, 23, 24, 25, 26, 27, 28, 30, 31, 33, 34, 35, 36, 37, 40, 42, 43, 44, 47, 48, 49, 54, 55, 56, 58, 60, 61, 62, 63, 64, 65, 66, 68, 70, 80, 90
protein aggregation, 2, 5, 15, 18, 37
protein degradation mechanism(s), vii, viii, 2, 11

protein modification, 8
proteins, vii, viii, 2, 4, 6, 7, 8, 10, 11, 14, 18, 19, 33, 40, 55, 58, 68, 78, 80
proteomic, 41, 67, 70

R

rats, viii, 18, 25, 28, 39, 46, 47, 54, 56, 57, 58, 63, 64, 65, 70, 91, 92
reactive nitrogen species, 4
reactive oxygen species, 4, 80
recirculation, 46, 47, 49, 53
recurrent stroke, 53, 67
redox regulation, vii, 1, 2, 35
regeneration processes, 51
reperfusion, 42, 49, 50, 51, 52, 53, 54, 58, 62, 64, 65

S

senile amyloid plaques, 46, 47, 54
serum, 18, 29, 49, 56, 61, 62, 68, 71
spatial memory, 53
striatum, 19, 49, 53
stroke, 33, 40, 41, 54, 56, 57, 58, 59, 60, 61, 62, 63, 67, 68, 69, 70, 71, 91, 93, 94
subarachnoid space, 53
subcortical white matter, 52
survival, 4, 26, 33, 42, 43, 44, 46, 47, 48, 49, 53, 64, 65, 66, 68, 83
synthase, 3, 8, 31, 34, 62

T

tau protein, viii, 17, 33, 40, 41, 47, 48, 49, 54, 55, 56, 57, 58, 61, 62, 67, 70
therapy, 25, 55, 65, 125, 139, 141
traumatic brain injury, ix, 73, 74, 76, 82, 83, 84, 85, 86, 87, 88

treatment, 17, 30, 40, 41, 57, 64, 75, 84, 97, 98, 114, 123, 136, 138, 139, 140, 141, 143
tremor, vii, x, 18, 95, 97, 98, 99, 100, 101, 102, 103, 117, 118, 119, 120, 121, 122, 123, 124, 125, 126, 136, 137, 138, 140, 141, 142, 143, 144, 145
tumor necrosis factor α, 51

U

unfolded protein responses (UPRs), 2, 3, 10, 36

W

white matter, viii, 39, 52, 65, 68, 69, 70, 82, 84
working memory, 53, 91

α

α-secretase, viii, 40, 43, 44, 54

β

β-amyloid peptide, 41, 47, 64, 65, 66
β-secretase, viii, 40, 42, 43, 44, 45, 54, 61, 66